Rapid Review of

ECG Interpretation

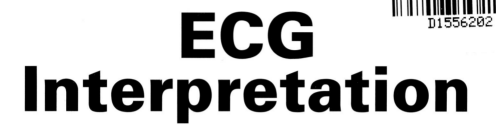

D1556202

Tariq Azeem
MBBS, MRCP
Specialist Registrar in Cardiology
Glenfield Hospital
Leicester, UK

Michael Vassallo
MD, FRCP, DGM, MPhil, PhD
Consultant Physician
The Royal Bournemouth Hospital
Bournemouth, UK

Nilesh J Samani
BSc, MD, FRCP, FACC, FMedSci
Professor of Cardiology
University of Leicester and Glenfield Hospital
Leicester, UK

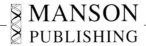
MANSON
PUBLISHING

For full details of all Manson Publishing Ltd titles please write to:
Manson Publishing Ltd, 73 Corringham Road, London NW11 7DL, UK.
Tel: +44(0)20 8905 5150
Fax: +44(0)20 8201 9233
Website: www.mansonpublishing.com

Commissioning editor: Jill Northcott
Project manager: Paul Bennett
Copy-editor: Ruth Maxwell
Designer: Alpha Media
Printed in India by Replika Press Pvt Ltd

Contents

Preface

The electrocardiogram (ECG) is a commonly used investigation in clinical practice. A working knowledge of the electrocardiogram is essential for the practising clinician. This book is intended as a succinct and enjoyable primer for junior doctors and students, including candidates preparing for both undergraduate and postgraduate examinations. The first section explains some of the basic principles of electrocardiography and includes a framework for the systematic evaluation of the ECG. Tables listing the differential diagnosis of common ECG abnormalities are provided. The second part of this book deals with more practical aspects of electrocardiography. By discussing 50 real case histories that illustrate all the major ECG abnormalities, it is hoped a more practical approach to learning the ECG is provided.

Tariq Azeem
Michael Vassallo
Nilesh J Samani

Abbreviations

ACC/AHA   American College of
   Cardiology/American Heart Association
AF   atrial fibrillation
ALT   alanine amino transferase
AP   anteroposterior
ASD   atrial septal defect
ATP   adenosine triphosphate
AV   atrioventricular
AVNRT   atrioventricular nodal re-entrant
   tachycardia
AVRT   atrioventricular re-entrant tachycardia
BBB   bundle branch block
BP   blood pressure
bpm   beats per minute
CCU   coronary care unit
CK/CKMB   creatinine kinase/creatinine kinase
   MB fraction
CSH   carotid sinus hypersensitivity
CSM   carotid sinus massage
CSS   carotid sinus syndrome
CT   computed tomography
CXR   chest X-ray
ECG   electrocardiogram
FBC   full blood count
Hb   haemoglobin
ICD   implantable cardiac defibrillator
K^+ potassium ion

L   left
LAD   left axis deviation
LDH   lactate dehydrogenase
LFT   liver function tests
LGL   Lown–Ganong–Levine (syndrome)
LVH   left ventricular hypertrophy
MCV   mean cell volume
MI   myocardial infarction
Na^+ sodium ion
NSTEMI   non-ST elevation myocardial infarction
QTc   corrected QT interval
R   right
RAD   right axis deviation
RV   right ventricle
RVH   right ventricular hypertrophy
SA   sinoatrial
STEMI   ST segment elevation myocardial
   infarction
SVT   supraventricular tachycardia
TFT   thyroid function tests
TSH   thyroid stimulating hormone
U&E   urea and electrolytes
VQ (scan)   ventilation perfusion (scan)
VSD   ventricular septal defect
VT   ventricular tachycardia
WPW   Wolff–Parkinson–White (syndrome)

Section 1
Principles of electrocardiography

Explaining the terminology
The electrodes

The ECG is recorded by applying electrodes to the limbs and to different parts of the praecordium. There are four limb and usually six chest electrodes (V1–V6). Occasionally additional chest electrodes are used to obtain more information regarding the right ventricle and posterior aspects of the heart. The position of the commonly used electrodes is given in *Table 1*. These positions are standardized and are shown in (**1**) and (**2**). These electrodes are used to generate the leads.

Table 1 Standard positions of the electrodes

Electrodes	Standard position
Limb	R arm
	L arm
	R leg (earth)
	L leg
Chest	
V1	4th intercostal space, just right of the sternum
V2	4th intercostal space, just left of the sternum
V3	Mid-way between V2 and V4
V4	5th intercostal space in the mid-clavicular line
V5	At the same level as V4 in the anterior axillary line
V6	At the same level as V5 in the mid-axillary line
Optional leads	
V7	At the same level as V6 but in the posterior axillary line
V3R	Equivalent position of V3 on the right side
V7R	Equivalent position of V7 on the right side

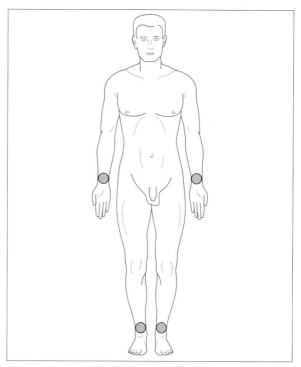

1 Position of limb electrodes.

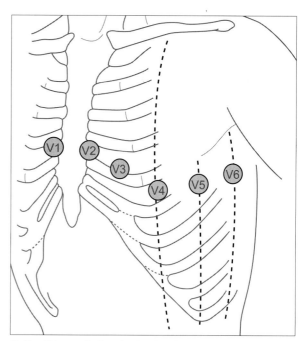

2 Position of chest electrodes.

The leads

An important concept to understand is that the leads assess the heart's electrical activity from particular viewpoints and should not be confused with the electrodes or connecting wires that record this electrical activity. A lead is obtained from two electrodes attached to the body. One of the electrodes is labelled as positive and the other negative. The imaginary line joining the two electrodes is the lead axis. For any electrical activity in the heart, the deflection in that lead will point upwards if the overall balance of the activity is moving towards the positive terminal and downward pointing if it is moving away from the positive terminal. There are two types of leads: the limb leads and the chest leads.

The limb leads

The limb leads assess the electrical activity of the heart in the frontal plane. There are six limb leads: LI, LII, LIII, aVR, aVL, and aVF. The positive and negative terminals of the common leads are given in *Table 2* and their relation to each other is shown in (**3**) and (**4**).

The LI, LII, and LIII leads are referred to as *bipolar* leads as they *directly* assess the activity between two of the limb electrodes. LI measures the potential difference between the right and left arms, LII between the right arm and the left leg, and LIII between the left leg and left arm.

The aVR, aVL, and aVF leads are referred to as unipolar leads, although they still measure the electrical activity between two terminals. However, in their case, the negative terminal (referred to as the central terminal) is made up of the sum of the electrodes attached to the right arm, left arm, and left leg. The sum of these three limb electrodes is at all times equal to zero potential. The voltage using this method is rather low and therefore needs to be augmented, hence the term 'augmented' or 'a' unipolar leads.

The chest (precordial) leads

The chest electrodes generate the chest leads V1, V2, V3, V4, V5, and V6. The chest leads measure the potential between these electrodes and the central terminal. These view the heart in the horizontal plane (**5**).

By convention, the standard ECG is composed of the above 12 leads so that all ECGs have the same format wherever they are recorded. However, additional electrodes can be used to view other areas of the heart, such as the right ventricle (V3R) or posterior surface of the heart (V7, V8, V9) (**5**).

One should now be able to understand the anatomical relationship of the ECG leads to the heart and the terms used in interpreting the ECG. The inferior leads are LII, LIII, and aVF because they look at the heart from the inferior aspect. The lateral leads are LI and aVL. The anterior leads are V1–V6, which are often further divided into anteroseptal (V1–V4) and lateral (V5–V6). V1 and V3R (if recorded) assess the right ventricle.

Table 2 The positive and negative terminals of the limb leads

Bipolar limb leads (frontal plane)

Lead I	R arm (-) to L arm (+)
Lead II	R arm (-) to L foot (+)
Lead III	L arm (-) to L foot (+)

Augmented unipolar limb leads (frontal plane)

Lead aVR	R arm (+) to common terminal (-)
Lead aVL	L arm (+) to common terminal (-)
Lead aVF	L foot (+) to common terminal (-)

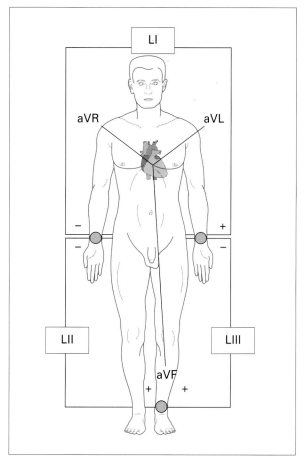

3 The limb leads of the ECG.

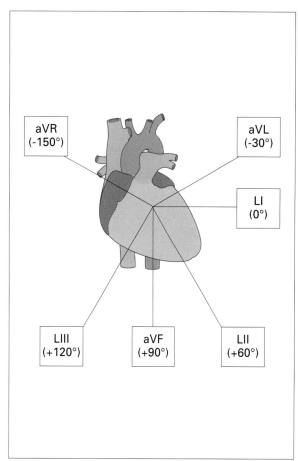

4 The view point each limb lead has of the heart.

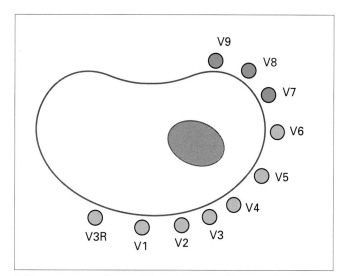

5 Transverse view of the chest and heart showing the relationship of the chest leads to each other.

The P-QRS-T complex

Action potential

The P-QRS-T complex (**6**) is generated through the propagation of an action potential through the cardiac cells (**7**). At rest the cell has a negative potential primarily due to the activity of the sodium pump, which extrudes positively charged Na^+ ions from the cells. A slight reduction in the resting potential due to the imminent arrival of the action potential from an adjacent cell results in a transient large increase in permeability for Na^+ ions and abrupt depolarization. This is followed by an active two-phase process of repolarization, during which the Na^+ ions are again actively extruded from the cells to restore the resting potential. During part of the repolarization phase the cell is refractory to further stimulation. In the meantime, the depolarization wave has moved to the next cell. The electrical impulse is usually generated in the sinoatrial (SA) node, which has specialized cells that spontaneously depolarize. The rate of depolarization of these cells is controlled by neural input from the sympathetic and vagal nerves.

The cardiac conducting system

When an electrical impulse is generated by the SA node it moves through the cardiac conducting system. The conduction system is a network of modified cardiac muscle cells that transmit the cardiac impulse through the vascular myocardium in a manner that ensures the synchronized action of the heart. A diagram of the components of the conduction system is shown in (**8**). The P-QRS-T complex is generated as the electrical impulse is conducted down this system.

The impulse starts by depolarization of the SA node. This event is too weak to register on the surface ECG. The impulse then travels through the atria via the internodal tracts, depolarizing them and generating a P wave on the surface ECG. The impulse reaches the atrioventricular (AV) node in the atrioventricular junction. There is a delay in the conduction of the impulse at this point contributing to the PR interval.

The impulse then travels down the atrioventricular bundle of His to reach the ventricles. In the normal heart the atria and the ventricles are well insulated by fibrous tissue to ensure that the only way electrical impulses travel down to the ventricles is through this route.

The bundle of His divides into right and left bundle branches that depolarize the right and left ventricles respectively. The left branch further divides into anterior and posterior branches. The depolarization of the ventricles produces the QRS complex. After the ventricular muscles are depolarized there is a time period where they cannot respond to further electrical stimuli. This is the refractory period. This can be absolute when there can be no response no matter how strong the stimulus, or relative when there can be a response to a stronger than normal stimulus. This refractory period is represented on the ECG by the ST segment. The muscle subsequently repolarizes to revert to its resting electrical state. This process is represented by the T wave. The U wave represents the period of greatest excitability of the ventricles. Its origin is unclear but it may represent the repolarization of the interventricular septum or the slow repolarization of the ventricles. Note that atrial repolarization is not normally visible because it is submerged in the QRS complex.

Components of the P-QRS-T complex

The normal ECG (**6**) therefore comprises a P wave, QRS complex, ST segment, and T wave. There may be another terminal deflection termed the U wave. A summary of the cardiac events generating the components of the ECG complex is given in *Table 3* (see page 10).

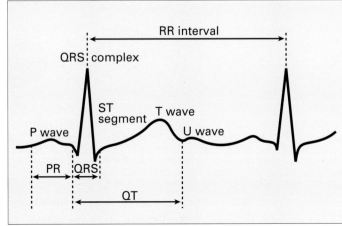

6 The components of the normal ECG.

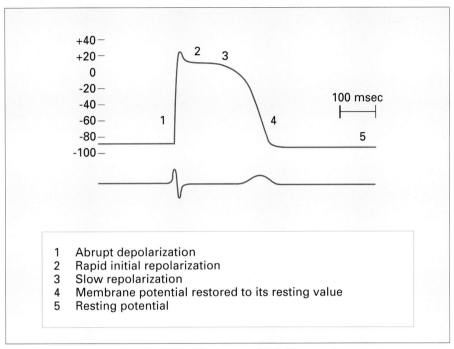

1 Abrupt depolarization
2 Rapid initial repolarization
3 Slow repolarization
4 Membrane potential restored to its resting value
5 Resting potential

7 The action potential and its relation to QRS-T complex.

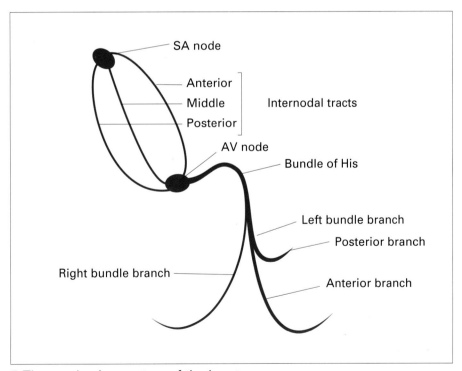

8 The conducting system of the heart.

Table 3 ECG reference points with corresponding cardiac events

ECG reference point	Cardiac event
P wave	Depolarization of the atria. Atrial repolarization is normally submerged in the QRS complex and is usually not visible
PR interval	Time from start of atrial depolarization to start of ventricular depolarization
QRS complex	Ventricular depolarization
ST segment	Time from end of ventricular depolarization to start of ventricular repolarization
T wave	Ventricular repolarization
QT interval	Total time of ventricular depolarization to repolarization
U wave	Origin is uncertain. It may represent the repolarization of the interventricular septum, or the slow repolarization of the ventricles, or the slow repolarization of the intraventricular conduction system

The 12 lead ECG

As explained earlier, each lead assesses the cardiac electrical activity from a particular viewpoint. As the electrical impulse moves towards a lead it generates a positive or upward deflection, and as it moves away the deflection is negative or downward. The configuration of the P-QRS-T wave in a lead is determined by the position of the lead in relation to this electrical activity (**9**).

The size of the potential recorded depends on the bulk of the structure being depolarized. In the normal ECG the P wave is smaller than the QRS complex as the atria are smaller than the ventricles. In addition the left ventricle is thicker than the right and the voltage generated when it depolarizes usually determines the size of the QRS complex.

A convention is applied to the description of the QRS complex. Large deflections are labelled as Q, R, and S while small deflections are labelled in lower case as q, r, and s. If the first deflection is downwards it is called a Q or q. The first positive deflection is labelled r or R, whether it is preceded by a Q or not. Any deflection below the baseline following an R wave is called an s or S wave whether there has been a preceding Q or not. Any second positive wave is labelled r' or R'. Any wave which is entirely negative is labelled as qs or QS.

Limb leads

Figure (**10**) illustrates the appearance of the P-QRS-T complexes in the limb leads. Rather than trying to remember the appearance of the various leads in the ECG, it is better to try to understand why the leads appear the way they do. As an aide memoire to do this one must remember the anatomical alignment of the conducting system and the depolarization process in relation to the anatomical position of the leads demonstrated in (**9**) and (**10**). Once the impulse reaches the interventricular septum it spreads from the left side of the septum towards the right ventricular cavity. It then spreads through the walls of the ventricles simultaneously from the endocardial to the epicardial surface. The left ventricle is significantly bulkier than the right ventricle and therefore the voltage generated by it will dominate the QRS complex. The direction and the size of the deflections generated in the ECG by this sequence of depolarizations depend on where the leads are placed and the direction of the impulse in relation to the lead as explained previously. In (**9**) the thicker the arrow the stronger the depolarization potential.

Bipolar leads

In LI and LII the electrical activity associated with atrial depolarization is moving towards the leads, resulting in upright P waves. The bulk of electrical activity associated with ventricular depolarization is

9 The flow of electrical activity in the heart and sequence of depolarization of the ventricles.

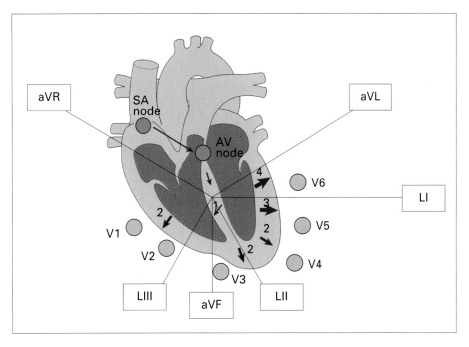

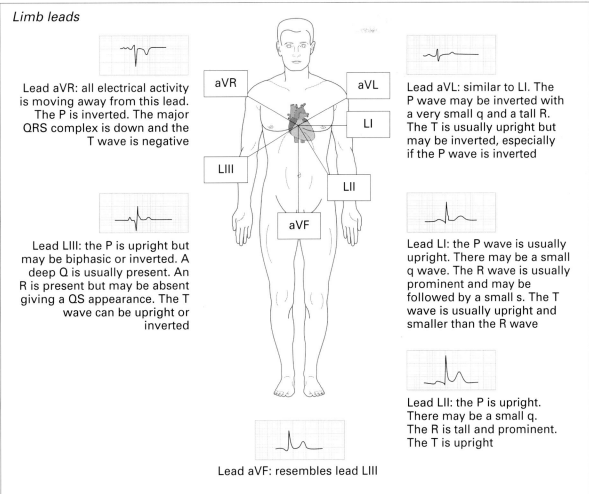

Limb leads

Lead aVR: all electrical activity is moving away from this lead. The P is inverted. The major QRS complex is down and the T wave is negative

Lead aVL: similar to LI. The P wave may be inverted with a very small q and a tall R. The T is usually upright but may be inverted, especially if the P wave is inverted

Lead LIII: the P is upright but may be biphasic or inverted. A deep Q is usually present. An R is present but may be absent giving a QS appearance. The T wave can be upright or inverted

Lead LI: the P wave is usually upright. There may be a small q wave. The R wave is usually prominent and may be followed by a small s. The T wave is usually upright and smaller than the R wave

Lead LII: the P is upright. There may be a small q. The R is tall and prominent. The T is upright

Lead aVF: resembles lead LIII

10 Limb leads: appearance of the leads in the normal ECG.

moving towards the leads, resulting in a prominent R wave in both these leads. One can find a small Q or S waves due to a smaller amount of electrical activity moving away from the leads, associated with septal and right ventricular depolarization. The T waves are usually upright in both leads. In LIII some electrical activity associated with atrial depolarization is moving away from the lead. The P wave may therefore be biphasic or inverted. The depolarization of the left ventricle is moving away from the lead and this results in deep Q or QS waves and inverted T waves. These waves must therefore be regarded as physiological if occuring in this lead alone. A deep Q and inverted T in LIII are abnormal only if present in other leads looking at the inferior surface of the heart, such as LII and aVF, or if there are reciprocal changes in LI and aVL. This lead may be affected by diaphragmatic movement causing variable Q and T waves changes. A smaller amount of electrical activity associated with septal and right ventricular depolarization is moving towards the lead, usually resulting in a small R wave.

Unipolar leads

In aVR all the electrical activity is moving away from the lead, resulting in negative P-QRS-T waves. Lead aVL is positioned close to L1 and there is close resemblance in the appearance of both leads. Some electrical activity associated with atrial depolarization moves away from the lead that may result in inverted P waves. AVF is close to LIII resulting in a similar appearance of both leads.

Chest (precordial) leads

In V1 there is a small R and a deep S wave. This is because from the view point of V1 only a smaller proportion of the electrical activity depolarizing the R ventricle is moving towards it (producing a small positive deflection, the R wave, while the bulk of the electrical activity is moving away to the left to depolarize the left ventricle, producing the negative larger S wave). As we move along to V6 the R wave becomes taller and the S wave shorter. This is because leads to the left of the chest have the bulk of the electrical current moving towards them producing a positive deflection (**11**).

Chest leads

P wave: P waves decrease in size from right to left. In V1 and V2 they are often inverted or biphasic. In the other leads they are upright.

QRS-complex: the r wave is small in V1 and increases in size as one moves from V1 to V6. The S wave shows a reverse trend. The R and S waves are approximately equal in size in V3 and V4. The initial direction of QRS complexes is positive in V1, V2, and V3 (r wave) and is negative in V4, V5, and V6 (q wave). This is due to initial septal depolarization (from left to right) and is only a small deflection. The leads V1–V3 show dominant S wave while leads V4–V6 show R wave. This is due to left ventricular depolarization which represents the bulk of depolarization action potential. The zone of change is called the transition zone. Normally, the transition zone lies between V3 and V4 (over the interventricular septum). Therefore leads V1–V3 lie over the right ventricle and leads V4–V6 lie over the left ventricle. The transition zone can be rotated in a clockwise or anticlockwise direction as explained later in axis deviation around the vertical axis (see page 18).

T wave: T waves are usually upright in all the chest leads although they may be inverted in V1 and V2.

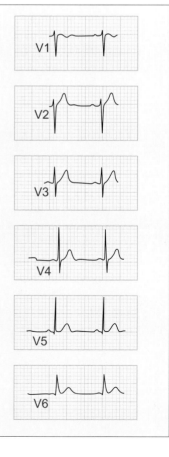

11 Chest leads: diagram demonstrating V1–V6.

Section 2
Comprehensive assessment
of the ECG

A comprehensive assessment of the electrocardiogram (ECG) requires a systematic approach. A cursory look can often miss important diagnoses. Each component of the ECG requires a separate analysis, and a routine is recommended. A suggested routine is given in *Table 4*.

It is essential to record the name, date, and time on every ECG. This ensures that the ECG can be a useful reference point when reviewed at any time in the future. Before analysing the ECG it is good practice to check these details. The ECG should be inspected for quality including any interference from skeletal muscle depolarizations (e.g. in a shivering patient) or mains frequency interference. When old ECGs are available compare them to the most recent. This is important in determining the diagnosis and deciding whether abnormalities are recent developments or old changes.

An initial assessment of rate, rhythm and axis is important. One can then proceed to look at the various components of the ECG in a systematic fashion. A logical way of doing this is by following the sequence of the ECG itself.

Rate

The ECG paper is composed of 1 mm and 5 mm squares (**12**). The machine is standardized that an impulse of 1 mV causes a deflection of 10 mm. The paper usually moves at a rate of 25 mm/second. One small square represents 0.04 seconds and a large square (5 mm) represents 0.2 seconds. When normal values are quoted they are based on this standard speed.

Table 4 Systematic assessment of the ECG

Step	Measure
1	Check name, time, and location where the ECG was performed
2	Compare the current ECG to previous ECGs if available
3	Determine rate, rhythm, and axis
4	P wave
5	PR interval
6	Q wave and QRS complex
7	ST segment
8	T wave
9	U wave

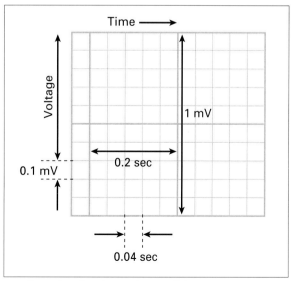

12 Standardization of the ECG.

Calculating the heart rate

If the heart rate is regular a simple way to calculate the rate quickly is to divide 300 (number of 5 mm squares in 1 minute) by the number of 5 mm squares between two QRS complexes.

This method cannot be used when the heart rate is irregular. In this case count the number of QRS complexes in 30 large squares (the number of beats in 6 seconds) and multiply by 10.

The normal resting heart rate ranges from 60–100 beats per minute. Common examples of rhythm abnormalities based on origin are given in *Table 5*.

Rhythm

To determine the rhythm accurately one needs to examine a rhythm strip. This is a prolonged recording of one lead (usually lead LII where P wave activity is best seen). A rhythm can be generated by the various structures of the heart (*Table 5*).

The normal cardiac rhythm is sinus rhythm. The SA node acts as the natural pacemaker and characteristically discharges impulses regularly at a rate of 60–100 times per minute. Abnormal cardiac rhythms can be subclassified as regular/irregular or bradycardia/tachycardia, depending on their characteristics.

The cardiac axis

The cardiac axis is a measure of the electrical position of the heart. The heart can rotate around an anteroposterior (AP) axis causing a left or right axis deviation, or a vertical axis causing a clockwise or anticlockwise rotation. It is important to note that the electrical position of the heart can change if there are changes in the anatomical position of the heart due to extrinsic factors (e.g. lung pathology). However, axis changes can also reflect cardiac abnormalities.

Table 5   Common examples of rhythm abnormalities based on origin

Sino-atrial (SA) node
- Normal: heart rate 60–100 bpm
- Sinus tachycardia: heart rate >100 bpm
- Sinus bradycardia: heart rate <60 bpm
- Sinus arrhythmia (**ECG 44**)
- Sinus node exit block

Atrio-ventricular (AV) node
- First degree heart block (**ECG 35a,** lead LII)
- Second degree heart block – it can subdivided into:
  – Mobitz type I (Wenckebach) heart block (**ECG 21**)
  – Mobitz type II heart block (**ECG 15a**)
- Complete heart block (**ECG 15b**)
- AV junctional rhythm (**ECG 13**)
- AV nodal re-entrant tachycardia (AVNRT)

Atria
- Wandering atrial pacemaker (**ECG18**)
- Atrial flutter (**ECG 39a**)
- Atrial fibrillation (**ECG 33**)
- AV re-entrant tachycardia (due to accessory pathway like in WPW syndrome) (**ECG 40b**)

Ventricles
- Idioventricular rhythm
- Ventricular tachycardia (**ECG 22a**)
- Torsades de points (polymorphic ventricular tachycardia) (**ECG 49**)
- Ventricular fibrillation

The AP axis

The AP axis is measured using a horizontal line through the heart as a reference (**13**). By convention, angles below the line are positive (0° to +180°) and above are negative (0° to -180°). The axis of each component of the ECG complex can be calculated but most interest lies in the axis of the QRS complex. The normal QRS axis in the frontal plane is -30° to +90°.

Calculating the QRS axis

A precise way of calculating the axis using the hexial system is shown in (**13**). Note that this is in large part an extension of (**4**) and shows the electrical views that particular leads have of the heart and the inverse of these leads. Particular attention must be paid to whether the leads are positive or negative.

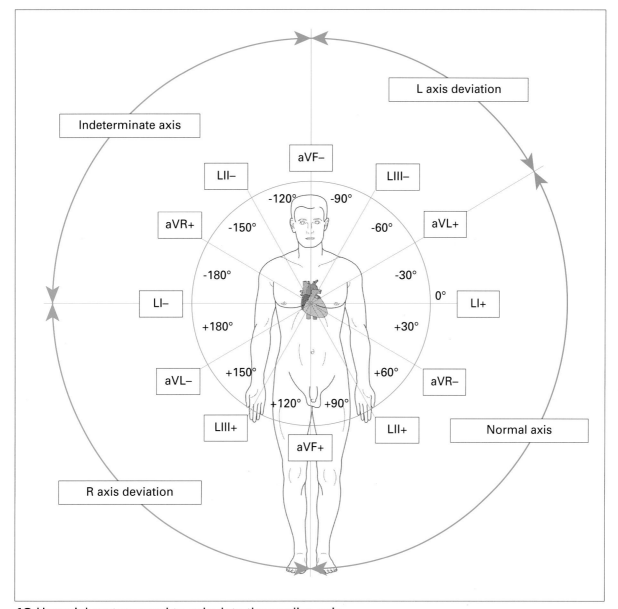

13 Hexaxial system used to calculate the cardiac axis.

To calculate the axis using this system one must go through four simple steps:

1 Identify the limb lead with the smallest and most equiphasic QRS deflection.
2 Look at the lead perpendicular to it and identify which is positive.

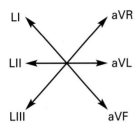

3 Now look at the hexaxial system. Read off the degrees from the positive or negative axis of the lead depending on whether the complex chosen in step 2 is positive or negative.
4 The last step is looking again at the lead chosen in stage 1. If this lead is exactly equiphasic no correction is needed to the value obtained in stage 3. If there is a small positive or negative deflection then the angle is a little bigger or smaller respectively.

Figure (**14**) is an example of how to calculate the axis.

A few simple rules

One can usually get an idea of the axis of the heart by looking at the QRS complex of leads LI/aVL and LIII/aVF.

• A left axis deviation is usually (but not necessarily) present when the main direction of the QRS complex in LI/aVL is up and diverges from the QRS complex in LIII/aVF which is down. Left axis deviation is especially likely if these changes are associated with a QRS complex in LII that has an S wave larger than the R wave.
• A right axis deviation is usually (but not necessarily) present when the main direction of the QRS complex points down in LI/aVL and up wards in LIII/aVF.
• A positive deflection in LI and LII is found with a normal axis.

Important causes of axis deviation are shown in *Table 6* and examples are illustrated in (**15**) and (**16**).

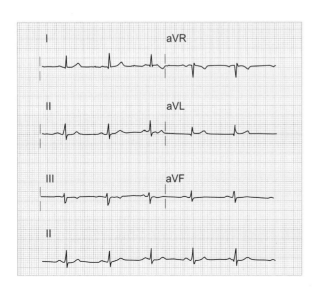

14 How to calculate the axis.
1 The smallest and most equal deflection is aVF.
2 The lead perpendicular to it is LI.
3 The deflection in LI is predominantly positive. From the hexaxial system, the positive end of LI is 0°.
4 Going back to aVF the deflection is not equiphasic and is more positive. A slight correction is therefore needed and the angle would be slightly smaller than 0°. The correction would be around +5°.

Table 6 Important causes of axis deviation

Axis and rotation
Normal -30° to +90°

L axis deviation <-30°
- L anterior hemiblock
- L ventricular hypertrophy
- WPW syndrome
- R ventricular ectopic beats
- Mechanical shift of the heart
- Normal in 10%
- ASD primum

R axis deviation >+90°
- Infancy
- Pulmonary embolism
- Normal variant
- Cor pulmonale
- ASD secundum
- R ventricular hypertrophy
- Some cases of R BBB
- L posterior hemiblock
- Dextrocardia
- L ventricular ectopic rhythm
- Congenital heart disease (Fallot's tetralogy)

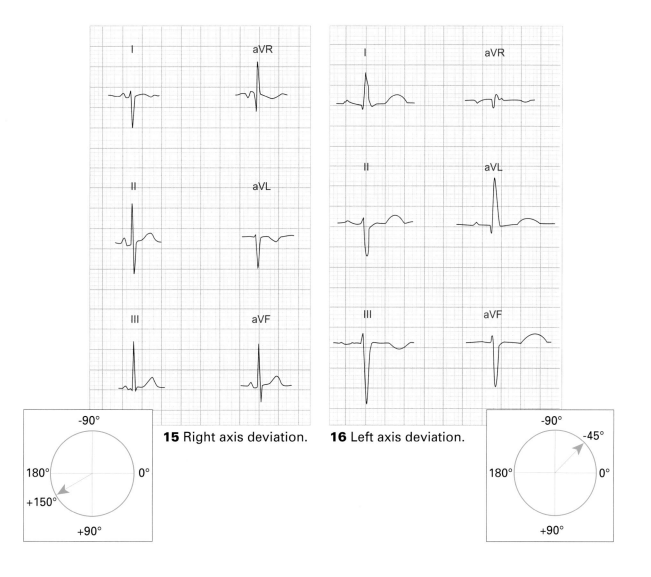

15 Right axis deviation.   **16** Left axis deviation.

Axis deviation around the vertical axis

The position of the heart around this axis is determined by examining the precordial leads, V1–V6. Moving from V1 to V6 one notices that the R wave progressively gets taller and the S wave shorter (**11**). Usually, the transition from a larger S to a larger R wave occurs at V3 or V4. This represents the normal position of the interventri-cular septum. If the R/S transition occurs at V5 or V6 then the heart is rotated clockwise. Conversely if the R/S transition occurs at V1 or V2 then the heart is rotated anticlockwise. Axis deviation in the vertical axis is usually not significant, by itself. The main concern is that the changes can mimic other diseases and in particular anterior myocardial infarctions. Examples of clockwise and anticlock-wise rotation are shown in (**17**).

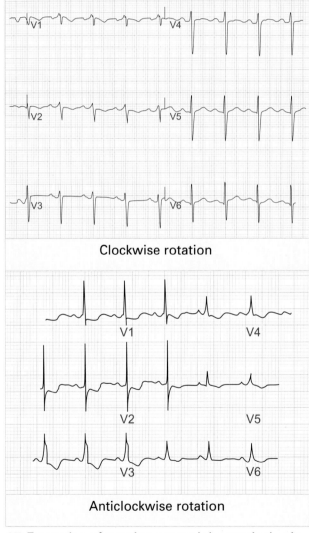

17 Examples of rotation around the vertical axis.

The P wave

The P wave is usually of low amplitude. It is upright in LI, LII, and LIII. Its height should not exceed 2.5 mm. The common types of P wave abnormalities are given in *Table 7*.

The PR interval

The PR interval represents the time taken for an impulse to travel through the AV node and bundle of His. It is measured from the beginning of the P wave to the beginning of the QRS complex. The normal PR interval is between 0.12–0.20 seconds, i.e. 3–5 small squares on a conventional ECG. The common types of PR interval abnormalities are given in *Table 8*.

Table 7   Common types of P wave abnormalities

Normal P wave
- Duration not >0.1 seconds (2.5 mm) and
- Height not >2.5 mm

Morphological abnormalities
- P mitrale (**ECG 11,** lead LII)
- P pulmonale (**ECG 20**)
- Wandering atrial pace maker

Multiple P waves per QRS complex
- Various degrees of AV blocks
- Atrial flutter with AV block

Absent P waves
- Atrial fibrillation
- AV junctional rhythm
- SA block

Inverted P waves
- Normal in some leads (e.g. aVR and V1)
- Wandering atrial pace maker
- AV junctional rhythm with retrograde conduction

Table 8   Common types of PR interval abnormalities

Normal PR interval
- Measured from the beginning of P wave to the beginning of QRS complex. It varies from 0.12 seconds to 0.2 seconds (3–5 mm)

Prolonged PR interval
- This is often referred to as first degree heart block and the PR interval is >0.2 seconds (>5 mm)

Short PR interval
- PR interval is <0.12 seconds (<3 mm). It may be a normal variant or a sign of accessory pathways, such as WPW syndrome

Variable PR interval
- A variable PR interval can be due to Wenckebach heart block, wandering atrial pace maker, or complete heart block

The Q (q) wave

A Q wave is present if the initial deflection of the QRS complex is downwards. Not all Q waves are pathological. The characteristics of normal and pathological Q (q) waves is shown in (**18**).

The QRS complex

The appearance of the normal QRS complex varies in different leads. Assessing whether any changes are pathological can be difficult and a useful way of doing this systematically is to assess whether the QRS complex appears wider, taller or smaller than expected, or has an abnormal shape. Based on this approach, (**19**) shows the characteristics of QRS complex abnormalities.

Normal
The duration is <0.04 seconds (1 mm), the depth is <2 mm in LI and LII (or <25% of the amplitude of the R wave) and 1 mm in any other lead. A deeper Q wave isolated in LIII may be a normal feature. This may be associated with an inverted T wave. Both disappear with deep inspiration

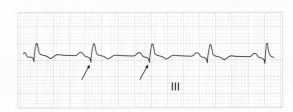

Abnormal
Q waves are pathological if they exceed the above criteria. This particular example is due to previous anterior wall MI. Further examples of Q waves are shown in Section 3

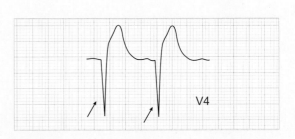

18 Characteristics of normal and pathological Q (q) waves.

19 Characteristics of QRS complex abnormalities.

Normal

The normal QRS duration is ≤0.10 seconds. QRS amplitude is quite variable from lead to lead and from person to person. It is determined by the size of the ventricular chambers (the larger the chamber, the larger the voltage) and proximity of the heart to the electrodes (the closer, the larger the voltage)

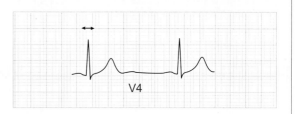

Widened QRS

The commonest abnormalities of widened abnormalities are due RBBB and LBBB. These are best seen in leads V1 and V6.

In RBBB there is rSR pattern in V1 and a terminal S wave with slurred upslope in V6.

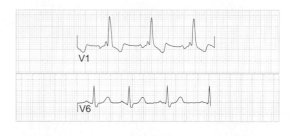

In LBBB there is M shaped QRS complex in V6

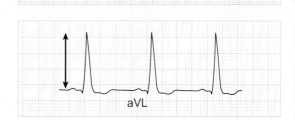

High voltage

The high voltage ECG can be due to ventricular hypertrophy or due to thin chest wall

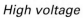

Low voltage

For low voltage ECG all the 12 leads should be seen because a low voltage QRS complex in an isolated lead may not have any significance. An important cause of low voltage ECG is cardiac tamponade due to pericardial effusion

Low voltage ECG in a patient with pericardial effusion. There is also electrical alternans in lead V5, that may be a sign of cardiac tamponade

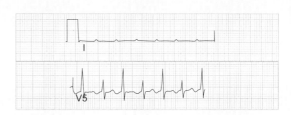

Abnormal shape

- Phasic aberrant ventricular conduction
- Acute pulmonary embolism
- Ventricular ectopics
- Ventricular tachycardia
- Ventricular fibrillation
- Torsades de points
- Electrical alternans
- Hyperkalaemia
- Changing axis deviation

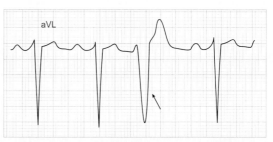

Ventricular ectopic

The ST segment

The ST segment represent the portion of the P-QRS-T complex between the end of the QRS complex (J point) and the beginning of the T wave. The ST segment is normally isoelectric. Therefore the main assessment of the ST segment relates to whether it is elevated or depressed. The common types of ST segment abnormalities are summarized in (**20**).

ST segment elevation

It is essential to note that not every ST segment elevation is pathological. Minor ST elevation in leads V–V3 may be normal, especially if large S waves are present. Such elevation is usually concave upwards and is not associated with any ST segment depression in the other leads. Similar elevation may also be seen in the other anterior leads. Normal ST elevation is referred to as 'high take off'.

The most important pathological cause of ST segment elevation is acute myocardial infarction (MI). When ST elevation is present there is transmural injury of the heart muscle. The ECG in ST

Elevation
- Physiological (high take off)
- Acute MI
- Pericarditis
- Cardiac trauma
- Hyperkalaemia
- Ventricular aneurysm

Depression
- Ischaemia
- Digitalis
- Ventricular strain
- Tachycardia
- Hypokalaemia
- Ventricular hypertrophy
- BBB
- Cardiomyopathy

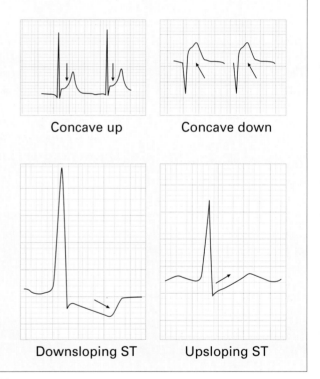

Concave up   Concave down

Downsloping ST   Upsloping ST

20 Common types of ST segment abnormalities.

segment elevation myocardial infarction (STEMI) evolves and changes over time. These changes are presented in (**21**). The appearance of the ECG may therefore help determine the approximate age of the infarct. A persistence of ST elevation post-MI may indicate the development of a ventricular aneurysm.

The other main pathological cause of ST elevation is acute pericarditis. ECG features that help to distinguish it from the ST elevation of an MI is that the changes are often widespread rather than localized to some leads (more typical of an MI) and the ST elevation is often concave up.

ST segment depression

ST segment depression can be upsloping or downsloping. The J point is the junction of the S wave and ST segment. During exercise upsloping ST depression is normal. The ST segment upslopes sharply and returns to the isoelectric line by 60 ms. Therefore, to assess for ST segment depression during exercise, one should always assess the ST segment at 80 ms (2 small squares) after the J point. Downsloping ST segment depression is always abnormal.

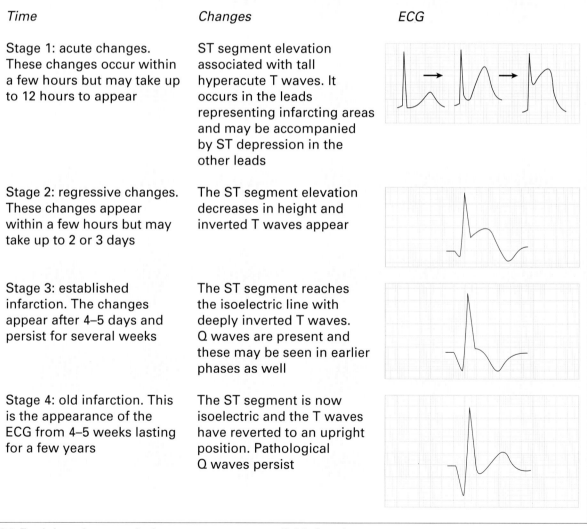

Time	Changes	ECG
Stage 1: acute changes. These changes occur within a few hours but may take up to 12 hours to appear	ST segment elevation associated with tall hyperacute T waves. It occurs in the leads representing infarcting areas and may be accompanied by ST depression in the other leads	
Stage 2: regressive changes. These changes appear within a few hours but may take up to 2 or 3 days	The ST segment elevation decreases in height and inverted T waves appear	
Stage 3: established infarction. The changes appear after 4–5 days and persist for several weeks	The ST segment reaches the isoelectric line with deeply inverted T waves. Q waves are present and these may be seen in earlier phases as well	
Stage 4: old infarction. This is the appearance of the ECG from 4–5 weeks lasting for a few years	The ST segment is now isoelectric and the T waves have reverted to an upright position. Pathological Q waves persist	

21 Evolving changes during an acute myocardial infarction.

The T wave

The T wave represents ventricular repolarization. A variety of factors can cause abnormalities of the T waves. The electrical basis of some of the abnormalities are not fully understood. Figure (**22**) shows the common types of T wave abnormalities.

The U wave

The U wave follows the T wave and is usually in the same direction as the T wave. It is not certain how the U wave originates although it is thought to be due to interventricular septum repolarization. It is not always present. Figure (**23**) shows the U wave.

Normal
No specified normal range. It is normally upright (except for leads aVR and V1), symmetrical, and usually is not more than half the size of the preceding QRS complex

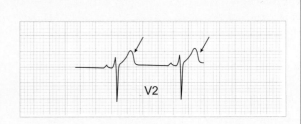

Tall
Hyperkalaemia is one of the important causes of tall T waves

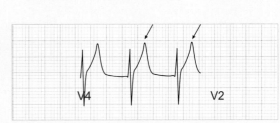

Flat
Important causes of flat T waves are:
* Physiological
* Myocardial ischaemia
* Hypothyroidism
* Pericarditis

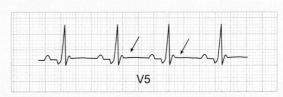

Inverted
Important causes of T wave inversion are:
* Myocardial ischaemia
* Non-ST elevation MI
* Pericarditis
* Hypokalaemia
* Ventricular hypertrophy
* Hyperventilation
* Physiological
* Complete heart block

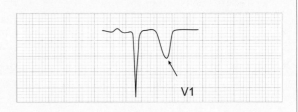

22 Common types of T wave abnormalities.

23 U wave.

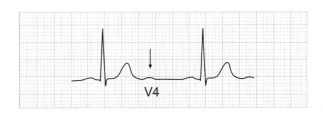

The QT interval

The QT interval is measured from the beginning of the QRS complex to the end of the T wave. This represents the total duration of electrical activity of the ventricles. If a U wave is present the QT interval is still measured to the end of the T wave. The QT interval is inversely related to cardiac rate. The faster the rate the shorter the QT interval and *vice versa*. Therefore, measurement of duration of QT intervals needs to take the heart rate into account. This corrected value of the QT interval is known as the QTc (corrected). Modern ECG machines are programmed to measure the QT interval and correct for heart rate automatically. However, the corrected QT interval can be worked out using Bazett's formula by dividing the observed QT interval in seconds by the square root of the RR interval in seconds:

$$QTc = \frac{\text{measured QT interval}}{\sqrt{\text{RR interval}}}$$

The normal QTc at a rate of 70 bpm does not exceed 0.40 seconds. For every 10 bpm increase above 70 bpm deduct 0.02 seconds and conversely for every 10 bpm below 70 bpm add 0.02. When the heart rate is 60 beats per minute the RR interval is 1 second. The √ RR interval (1 second) is 1 and the QTc is equal to the measured QT interval.

Variations in QT interval can indicate cardiac abnormalities and a prolonged QT interval can predispose to malignant ventricular arrythmias. Figure (**24**) shows the common types of QT interval abnormalities.

QTc dispersion is emerging as an important ECG measure. It represents the difference between the longest and shortest QTc interval in the different leads of an ECG. It is simple but time consuming to calculate manually. Increased QTc dispersion reflects inhomogeneity in ventricular repolarization. QTc dispersion of >60 ms has been reported to have a 92% sensitivity and 81% specificity of predicting cardiac death in patients following a heart attack or those with chronic heart failure.

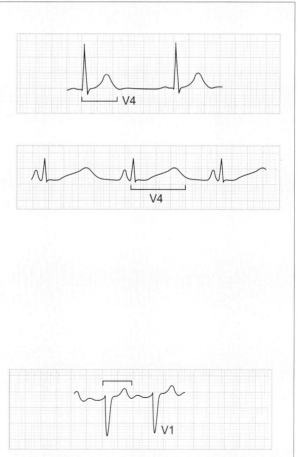

Normal
Measured from the beginning of the Q wave to the end of the T wave; the maximum duration is 0.4 seconds (10 mm) for a cardiac rate of 70 bpm

Prolonged QT
Important causes of prolonged QT interval are:
- Antiarrhythmic drugs, e.g. amiodarone, quinidine, flecainide
- Congenital
- Hypocalcaemia
- Hypokalaemia
  Drugs, e.g. neuroleptics, tricyclic antidepressants, antihistamines
- Ischaemic heart disease
- Carditis
- Cardiomegaly

Short QT
Impoprtant causes are:
- Digitalis
- Hypercalcaemia

24 Common types of QT interval abnormalities.

Section 3 Cases

Question 1

An 84-year-old male presented with sudden onset of chest pain. He was operated on for a fractured femur 10 days previously. He was cold, clammy, and hypotensive. He died on the following day after sustaining a cardiac arrest.

1 What are the findings in **ECG 1**?
2 What is the most likely diagnosis?

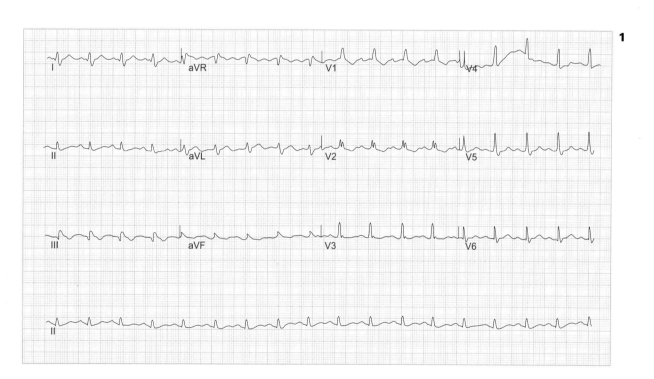

1

Answer 1

1 **ECG 1** shows sinus tachycardia (106 bpm), partial RBBB with an RSr pattern, and T wave inversion (circles) in leads V1 and V2 (right ventricular leads). There is also an 'S1 Q3 T3' pattern in limb leads LI and LIII (arrows).

2 These changes are consistent with the diagnosis of acute pulmonary embolism. Not all pulmonary emboli give rise to ECG changes. In addition the changes may be transient. The most common electro-cardiographic abnormality associated with pulmonary embolism is sinus tachycardia. Other features that may be seen, but are not present in this example, include right axis deviation, P pulmonale (best seen in leads LII and V1), and ST segment depression in leads V5 and V6. Rhythm changes can also occur. These include atrial or ventricular ectopics, AF, or supraventricular tachycardia (SVT). One should remember that none of these changes are specific for pulmonary embolism and the tracing should be interpreted in the light of the clinical presentation. This ECG and history strongly suggest the diagnosis of acute massive pulmonary embolism. This was confirmed on post mortem.

1
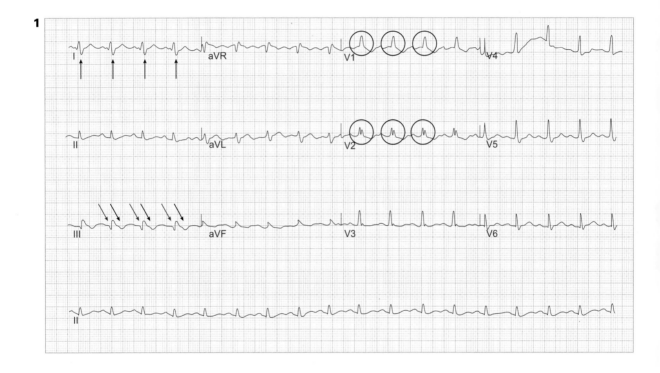

Question 2

A 61-year-old diabetic male presented with central crushing chest pain. **ECG 2a** was taken.

1 What are the findings in **ECG 2a**?
2 ECG 2b was taken after streptokinase was administered. What are the findings?
3 ECG 2c was taken from another patient. What are the findings?

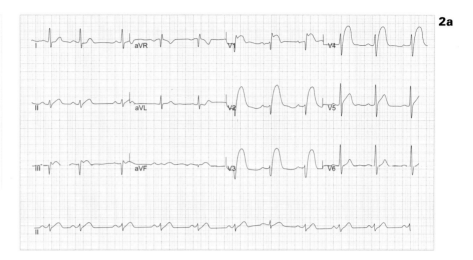

2a

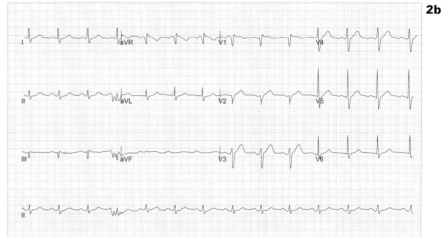

2b

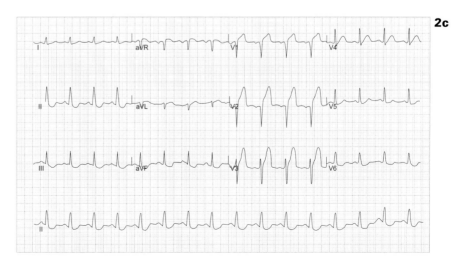

2c

Answer 2

1 ECG 2a shows sinus rhythm with first degree heart block (0.21 seconds) and a normal P-QRS complex. There is marked ST segment elevation in leads V1–V5 indicating acute anterior wall MI (arrows).

2 ECG 2b was taken after giving streptokinase. It shows complete resolution of the changes seen in the earlier ECG suggesting an excellent response to thrombolytic therapy. The cardiac enzymes were subsequently elevated, confirming the presence of myocardial damage.

3 ECG 2c shows sinus rhythm with ST segment elevation in leads V1–V3 (arrows) suggesting an acute anteroseptal MI. There are pathological Q waves visible in leads V1–V2 (circles). There is also ST depression seen in leads LII, LIII, aVF, and V6 (arrows), indicating inferolateral ischaemia.

2a

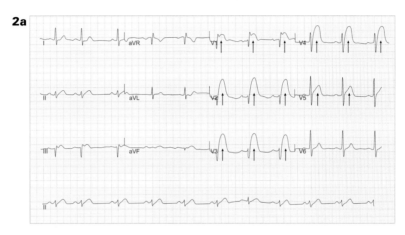

2b

2c

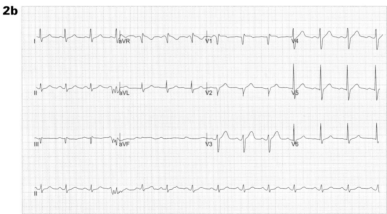

Question 3

A 43-year-old female presented with chest pain that became worse on inspiration. She had a recent history of a flu-like illness. **ECG 3a** was recorded on admission while **3b** was recorded 12 months later.

What are the findings in **ECG 3a** and what is the diagnosis?

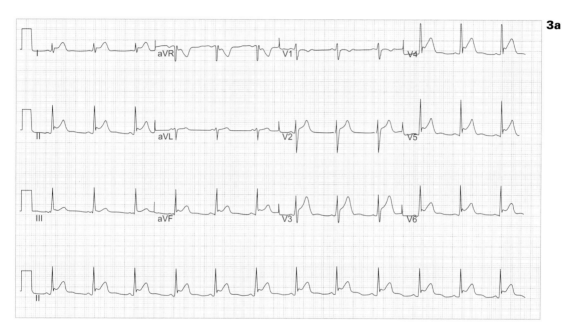

3a

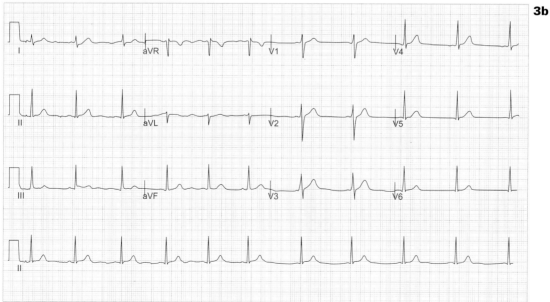

3b

Answer 3

ECG 3a shows sinus rhythm with generalized concave upwards ST segment elevation (arrows) across all the leads except aVL and V1. The morphology of the ST segment elevation and its widespread distribution indicates acute pericarditis. The ST segment elevation in pericarditis differs from acute ischaemia. It is concave upwards, unlike in acute MI when it is concave downwards. Furthermore, in acute MI the changes are limited to one particular segment supplied by a coronary artery, in contrast to pericarditis where the changes are widespread. More commonly, ECG changes in pericarditis are less specific and show T wave inversion only. With the development of a pericardial effusion the voltage falls and with large effusions electrical alternans may develop.

    ECG 3b shows complete resolution of the abnormalities associated with pericarditis in the earlier ECG.

3a

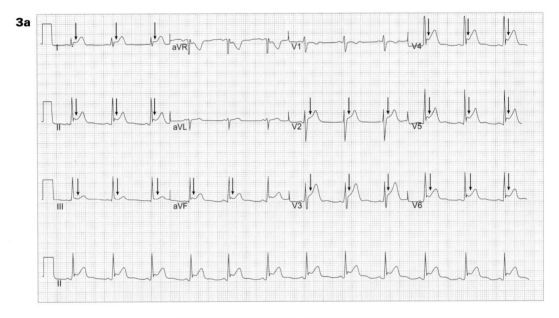

3b

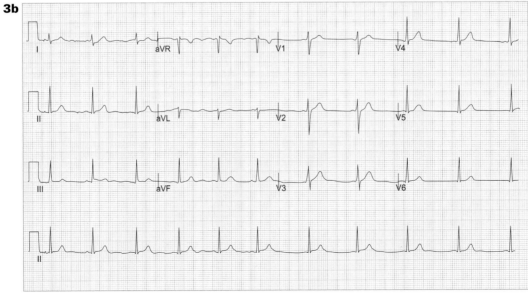

Question 4

A 52-year-old male who had MI 12 years previously, presented with exertional chest pain and shortness of breath. He had recurrent episodes of palpitations. Cardiac enzymes on admission were normal. **ECG 4** was performed while he was asymptomatic. An ECG a week later was identical.

1 What are the findings in **ECG 4**?
2 What is the diagnosis and what are the common presenting features of this condition?
3 How should the diagnosis be confirmed and what further investigation is appropriate?

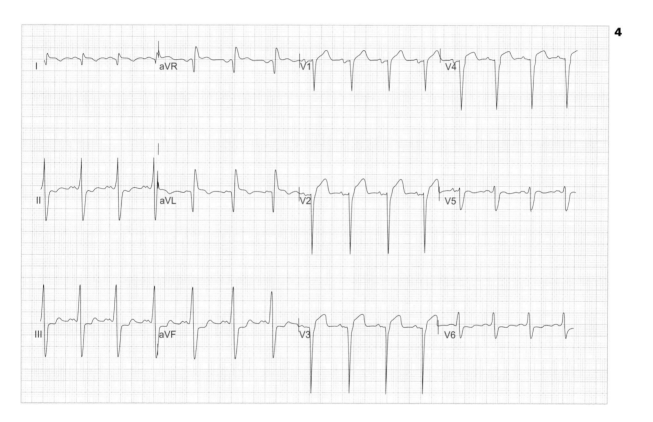

4

Answer 4

1 ECG 4 shows sinus rhythm. There are pathological Q waves in leads LI, aVL, and V1–V4. There is ST segment elevation in the same leads (arrows). There is also ST segment depression in leads LII, LIII, and aVF. There are bifid P waves in leads LII, LIII, and aVF (P mitrale; circles) indicating left atrial hypertrophy.

2 The above ECG changes and persistent ST segment elevation in the anterior chest leads over several years suggest the diagnosis of a ventricular aneurysm. Common presenting features of a ventricular aneurysm include intractable left ventricular failure with or without angina, angina alone, ventricular arrhythmias, and thromboembolism.

3 The diagnosis needs to be confirmed by echocardiography and/or ventriculography, since by no means all patients with persistent ST segment elevation on ECG have an aneurysm. A 24-hour ECG should be requested to rule out the possibility of serious dysrhythmias such as VT.

4

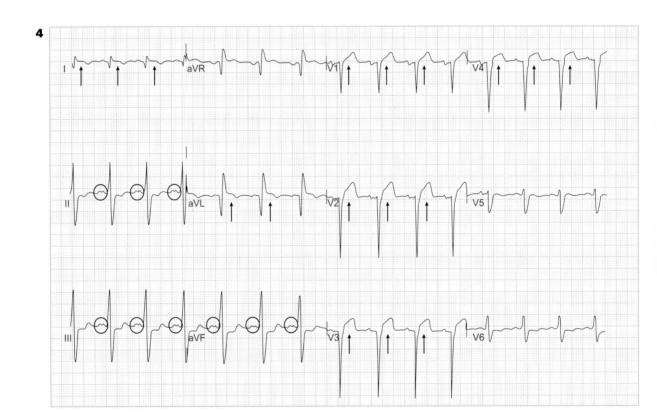

Question 5

A 75-year-old known hypertensive female was found to have **ECG 5** on routine examination.

What are the findings in **ECG 5**?

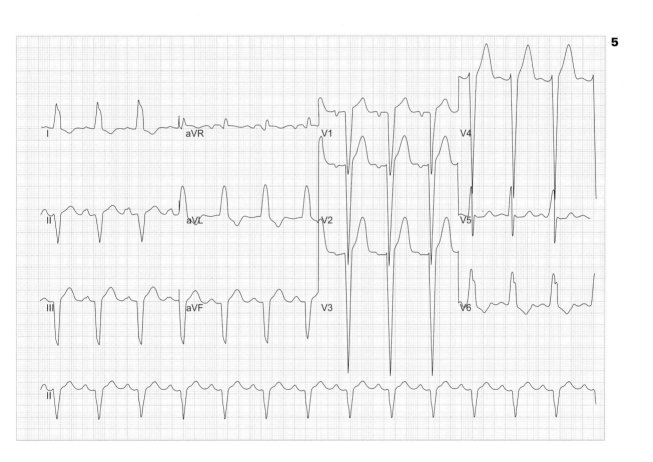

Answer 5

ECG 5 shows sinus rhythm with LAD. There are broad and bifid P waves (P mitrale) in leads LII, LIII, and aVF (circles). The QRS complex is prolonged in duration and M-shaped in LI and V6 (arrows), indicating the presence of complete LBBB.

The criteria for the diagnosis of LBBB include a total QRS duration of ≥0.12 seconds. The QRS complexes in the lateral leads (LI, aVL, and V5–V6) may be notched and tend to have an rsR or a broad monophasic R wave. Secondary T wave inversion and ST segment depression may be found in the left precordial leads and also in leads LI and aVL. The S waves in the right precordial leads are often abnormally deep. The initial R wave in the right precordial leads may be very small or absent. The mean frontal axis is usually in the normal range in uncomplicated cases, and abnormal LAD is not a routine feature of LBBB.

When LBBB is combined with an abnormal LAD, extensive disease of the left ventricular conducting tissue is likely to be present involving the peripheral part of the anterosuperior division of the left bundle branch system, as well as the proximal part of the left main bundle. When LBBB is combined with RAD, the possibility of coexisting RVH should be considered. In LBBB the early part of the QRS complex is involved due to an abnormal ventricular depolarization. It is therefore more difficult to diagnose MI in the presence of LBBB.

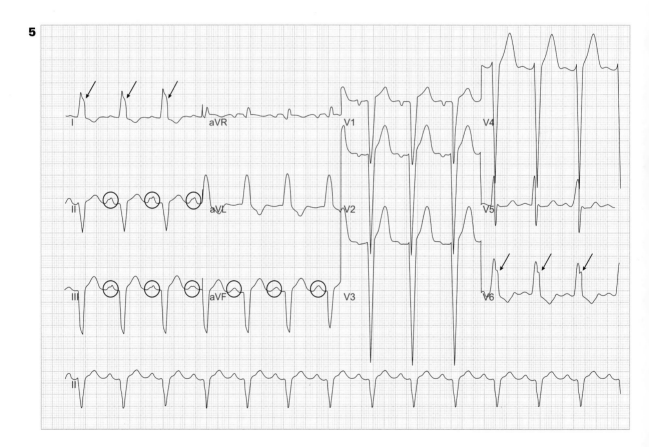

Question 6

An 87-year-old female presented with retrosternal, crushing chest pain associated with hypotension (BP 80/60 mmHg [10.7/8.0 kPa]) and a pulse of 23 bpm.

1 What are the findings in **ECG 6**?
2 How should this patient be managed?

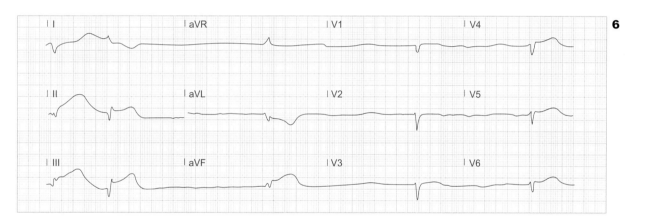

Answer 6

1 ECG 6 shows slow junctional escape rhythm with a ventricular rate of 23 bpm. There is ST segment elevation in leads LII, LIII, and aVF, with ST segment depression and T wave inversion in leads LI and aVL (arrows). The absence of P waves, the profound bradycardia, and the QRS complex of normal duration indicate junctional escape rhythm. The diagnosis is acute inferior wall MI, with lateral wall ischaemia and junctional escape rhythm.

The escape rhythm develops when there is cessation of pacemaker activity at the SA node. Any area in the conduction system starting from the AV node, His bundle, or any focus from within the ventricles may start discharging the impulses and take over as pacemaker.

Bradyarrhythmias are more common with inferior wall MIs. The inferior wall is supplied by the right coronary artery that also supplies the atria, right ventricle, and SA and AV nodes in the majority of cases (70–80%). Other bradyarrhythmias commonly associated with inferior wall MI are sinus bradycardia, sinus arrest, and AV blocks including complete heart block.

2 This patient requires urgent temporary pacing. Atropine intravenously or isoprenaline infusion may help as a temporary measure. If unsuccessful, external temporary pacing should be considered. The patient should also be considered for thrombolysis unless there are any contraindications.

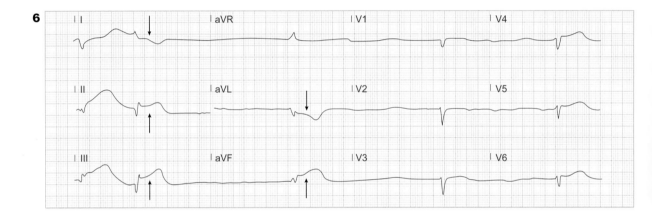

Question 7

A 40-year-old male who was a professional cyclist presented with sharp left-sided infra-mammary chest pain.

1 What are the findings in **ECG 7a**?
2 **ECG 7b** was taken after intravenous atropine. What does it show?

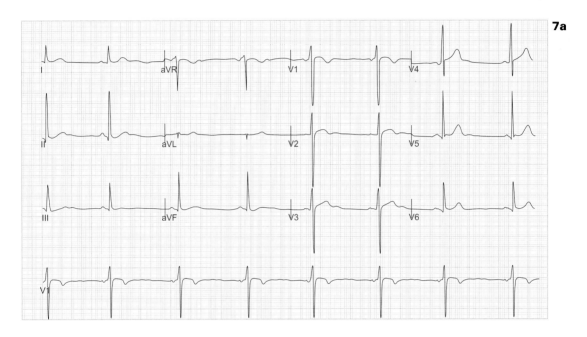

7a

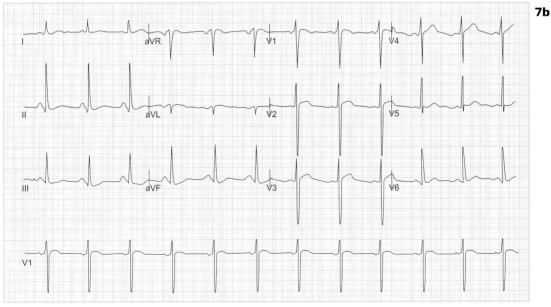

7b

Answer 7

1 ECG **7a** shows sinus bradycardia with a heart rate of 44 bpm. There is mild ST segment elevation in leads V2–V6 with U waves (arrows) visible in leads V2–V5. There is also LVH by voltage criteria (S wave in V2 and R wave in V5 is 47 mm, i.e. >35 mm confirming LVH). These are recognized electrocardiographic variations in trained athletes. Other electrocardiograpic features seen in athletes include sinus arrhythmia, first degree heart block, Wenckebach heart block, junctional rhythm, wandering atrial pacemaker, tall symmetrical T waves, and tall R waves. In marked sinus bradycardia there may be T wave abnormalities due to changes in repolarization, which may not necessarily represent ischaemic heart disease. These changes represent a high resting vagal tone in athletes.

2 On increasing the heart rate these changes disappear as seen in **ECG 7b** taken after giving 1.2 mg of atropine intravenously. This indicates the physiological nature of the changes. An alternative is to ask the patient to perform gentle exercise. However, both of these measures should be avoided in patients with a typical history of chest pain suggesting myocardial ischaemia, and in patients with already known coronary artery disease.

7a

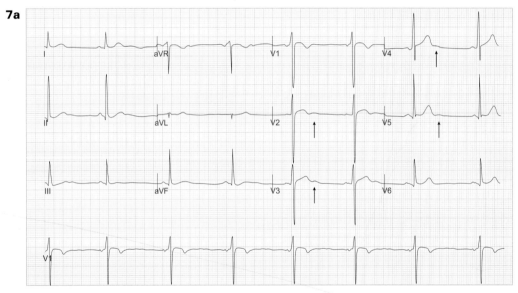

7b

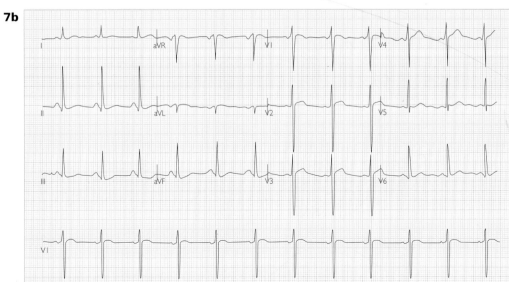

Question 8

ECG 8a was taken from a 76-year-old male who presented with palpitations and shortness of breath.

What are the findings in **ECG 8a**?

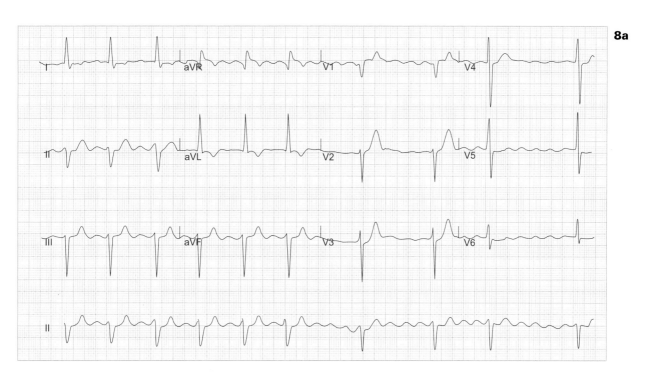

8a

Answer 8

ECG 8a shows atrial flutter with variable AV block. There is also LAD secondary to a left anterior hemiblock

In **ECG 8a** atrial activity is represented by the typical 'F' waves of atrial flutter (arrows) with the classical saw-tooth appearance occurring at a rate of 230 bpm. The atrial rate in patients with atrial flutter is usually around 300 bpm. The QRS complexes occurring at a rate of 60 bpm are of normal duration and are preceded by a variable number of F waves, ranging from 1–4. Atrial flutter is usually associated with organic heart disease, especially ischaemic and hypertensive heart disease. It may also occur in rheumatic heart disease and cor pulmonale. Initially, the arrhythmia may occur in discrete attacks but these become more persistent preceding the development of permanent AF.

In this case the atrial rate was slower than expected because the patient was on antiarrhythmic medication. Occasionally when the atrial rate is very rapid, the ECG shows a combination of flutter (F) and fibrillation (f) waves (arrows) as in **ECG 8b**. This is sometimes called flutter/fibrillation or impure flutter and usually progresses to AF. In elderly people there may be associated disease of the conducting tissue protecting the ventricle from a rapid ventricular rate.

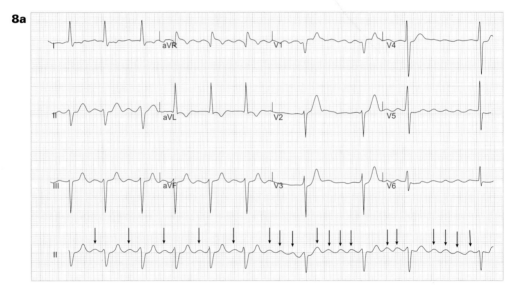

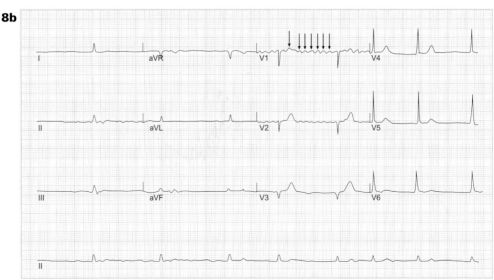

Question 9

An asymptomatic 75-year-old male was found to have **ECG 9** on a routine health check.

What is the differential diagnosis in **ECG 9**?

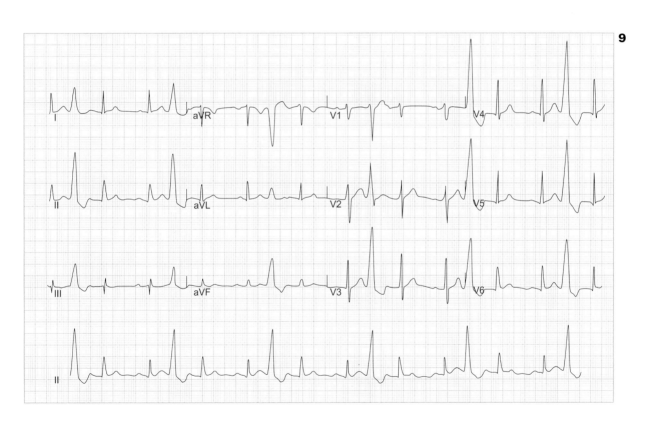

9

Answer 9

ECG 9 shows parasystole. This can occur in healthy individuals but more commonly occurs in the presence of severe organic heart disease. It is usually of little clinical significance and treatment is not usually warranted. It is a rhythm arising from an ectopic focus protected from being suppressed by the SA node (entrance block). It therefore imposes its own rhythm in addition to the rhythm arising from the SA node. The differential diagnosis would be ventricular trigeminy; however, the management of this condition would be the same.

There are four criteria before parasystole can be diagnosed. Firstly, since the parasystolic focus arises from a pacemaker not dependent on the dominant rhythm, there must be a variable coupling interval with the beats preceding them, unless the two rates have a common factor. Secondly, the interectopic intervals must be multiples of a common factor. Thirdly, the parasystolic cycle differs from the basic rhythm and is usually slower. Finally, because the ventricles may be activated by chance by both ectopic and normal pacemakers, fusion beats (complexes with the appearance of a combination of a normal and ectopic beat) may occur.

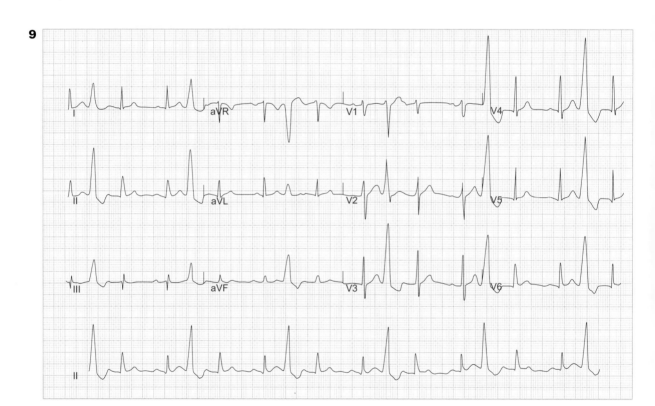

Question 10

An 80-year-old male who lives alone presented with a history of progressive confusion and drowsiness. He smelled of alcohol.

1 What are the findings in **ECG 10**?
2 Are the changes pathognomonic of the underlying condition?
3 What are the other arrhythmias associated with this condition?

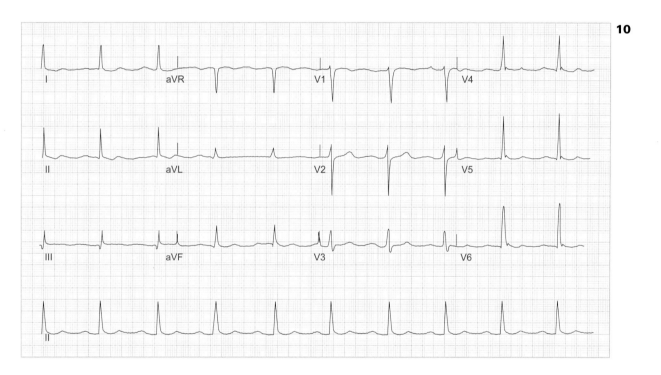

Answer 10

1 **ECG 10** shows sinus bradycardia with a normal axis. There is a prolonged PR interval indicating first degree heart block. The QRS complex has normal morphology but this is followed by a 'J' wave most prominently seen in leads V4–V6 (arrows). A J wave, also known as an Osbourne wave, is a deflection in the ECG appearing as a late delta wave or a small secondary r wave following the QRS complex. The QTc interval is prolonged to 452 ms.

2 This patient was found to be hypothermic with a temperature of 32°C (90°F). The J waves disappeared when the patient was slowly re-warmed. These are found in 80% of patients suffering from hypothermia. Generally the amplitude and duration are inversely related to core temperature. They have been described in normothermic patients with hypercalcaemia. Therefore, they should not be considered pathognomonic of hypothermia.

3 Other arrhythmias associated with hypothermia are sinus bradycardia, atrial fibrillation (AF) followed by ventricular fibrillation, and asystole. Prolonged resuscitation is recommended in hypothermia. The ventricular fibrillation is usually resistant to defibrillation if the core body temperature is <30°C (86°F).

10

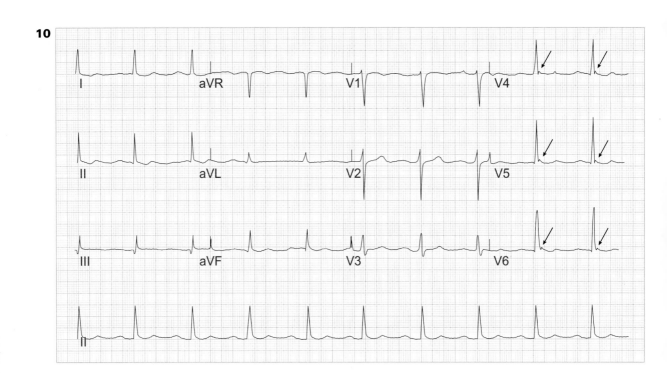

Question 11

A 75-year-old male presented with a history of chest pain and palpitations.

1 What are the findings in **ECG 11**?
2 What are the criteria for left atrial hypertrophy?

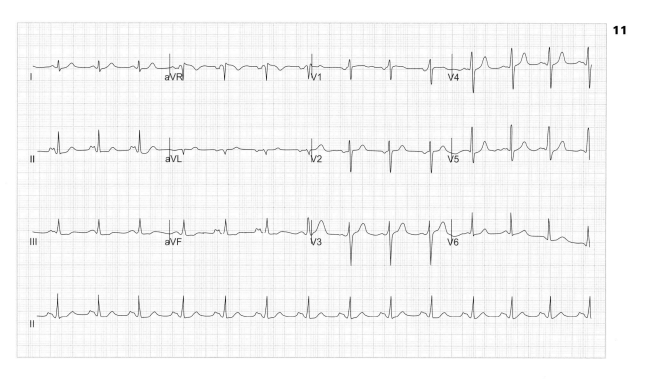

11

Answer 11

1 ECG 11 shows sinus rhythm. The axis is normal. There are broad M-shaped P waves seen most prominently in leads LII, LIII, and aVF (arrows).

2 In P mitrale the P waves are wide and bifid. The first peak represents right atrial activity and the second left atrial activity. The bifid P mitrale implies a delay in the activation of the left atrium. Criteria for left atrial hypertrophy include a P wave that is notched and exceeds 0.12 seconds in duration in leads LI, LII, aVF, or aVL. The P wave in lead V1 has a dominant negative component. It may be entirely negative or the terminal negative component may exceed the initial positive component. Left atrial hypertrophy usually occurs in association with left ventricular hypertrophy (LVH). The absence of LVH in this patient may indicate the presence of an underlying mitral stenosis. This was confirmed on echocardiography. Mitral stenosis can cause pulmonary hypertension leading to right ventricular hypertrophy (RVH) that may be seen concomitantly.

When interpreting abnormalities of the P wave one must remember that the P wave is less well defined than the QRS complex and consequently abnormalities of the P wave are less specific. Although the term hypertrophy is used very commonly, it is difficult to differentiate it from ischaemia, infarction, or conduction defects within the atrium. When clinical evidence of mitral stenosis or LVH is present, the presence of true left atrial hypertrophy can be inferred. However, if no such evidence is available, it can be difficult to determine the underlying aetiology.

11

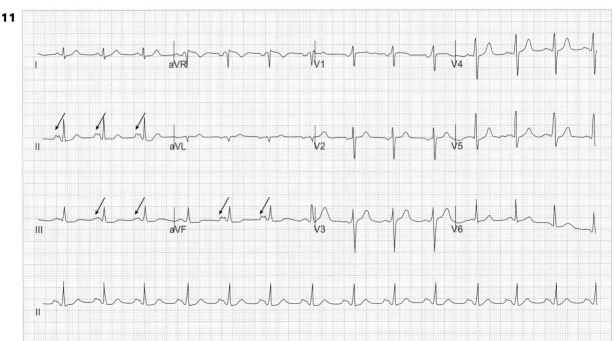

Question 12

A 40-year-old female presented with chest pain. She had no risk factors for coronary artery disease apart from a strong family history. Resting ECG and cardiac enzymes were within normal limits. A standard Bruce protocol exercise test was organized. **ECG 12** was taken at stage 1 of the exercise test.

1 What are the findings in **ECG 12**?
2 What do the findings suggest?

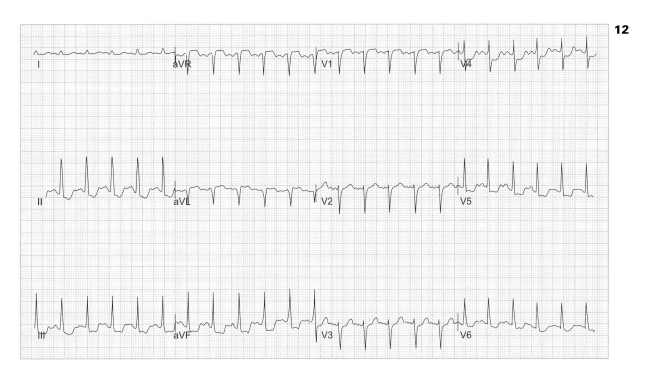

12

Answer 12

1 ECG 12 shows sinus tachycardia consistent with exercise. The P waves and QRS complexes are normal. However, significant extensive downsloping ST segment depression is seen in leads LII, LIII, aVF, and V4–V6 (arrows). A very important observation is that these changes occurred very early in this test at a low workload.

2 The ST segment depression is the most common manifestation of exercise-induced ischaemia. It is usually measured 80 ms (two small squares) after the J point, which is taken as the junction of the S wave and the ST segment. The ST segment depression should be considered significant if it is horizontal or downsloping and is ≥1 mm. Indicators of the probability of ischaemic heart disease in an exercise tolerance test are the occurrence of chest pain, the degree of ST segment depression, and the shortened duration of exercise.

The degree of ST segment depression and the low level of exercise at which changes appeared, suggests a very high probability of prognostically significant coronary artery disease. Various scores are used at exercise testing. They have been developed to determine prognosis and stratify risk. Such an example is the Duke score that measures exercise time and chest pain, in addition to ST segment depression.

12

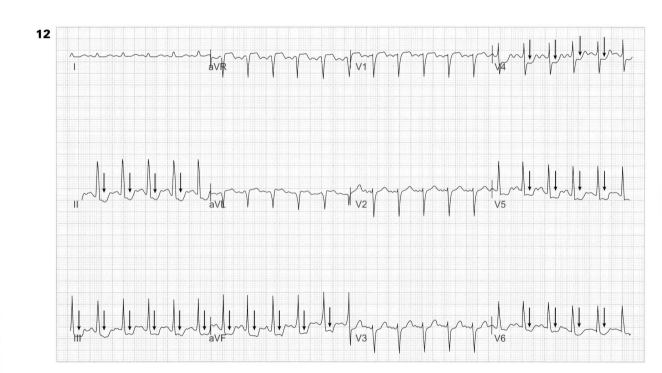

Question 13

A 79-year-old female without any significant past medical history presented with dizzy spells. She also had two blackouts with a spontaneous recovery. She was on no medication.

1 What are the findings on **ECG 13**?
2 How should this patient be managed?

13

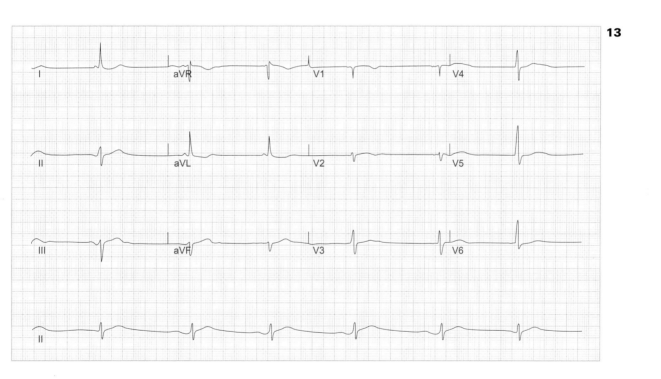

Answer 13

1 ECG 13 shows junctional escape rhythm with a rate of 39 bpm. The axis is normal. The P waves are visible just before the normal QRS complexes. They are of abnormal morphology. They are narrow, of low amplitude, inverted in LII and LIII, and are merging with the QRS complexes (arrows). P waves in junctional rhythm may be absent in the presence of a retrograde block. However, when present, the P waves are abnormal and usually of opposite polarity to normal P waves due to atrial activation in the opposite direction to normal. They may precede, coincide with, or follow the QRS complexes depending on the precise site of origin of the rhythm. The QRS complexes in this case are of normal morphology. The presence of abnormal P waves and normal QRS complexes suggests a high junctional origin. In escape rhythms lower than the AV junction, QRS complex duration is broadened.

The commonest cause for junctional rhythm is underlying myocardial ischaemia. It can also be due to medication such as digoxin, beta blockers, and rate-limiting calcium channel blockers such as verapamil and diltiazem.

2 With this background and current ECG the patient needs a permanent pacemaker.

13

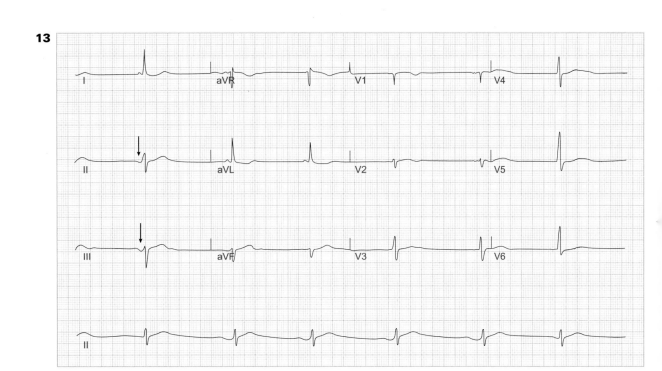

Question 14

This 33-year-old male presented with palpitations. **ECG 14a** was taken.

1 What are the findings in **ECG 14a**?
2 What are the common arrhythmias associated with this condition?
3 **ECG 14b** is from a different patient. What is the diagnosis?
4 What are the associations of this condition?

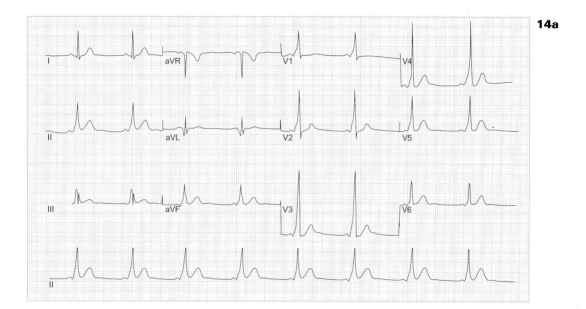

14a

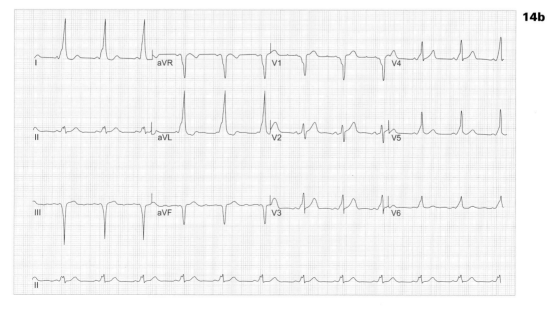

14b

Answer 14

1 ECG 14a shows a shortened PR interval with the presence of a positive delta wave (arrows) in lead V1–V5. This is characteristic of WPW type A syndrome. The delta wave is due to premature activation of the ventricle via an accessory pathway known as the bundle of Kent. The bundle of Kent is situated in the AV groove. If the pathway is situated in the left heart, the ECG is likely to show a positive delta wave in leads V1–V6 and a negative delta wave in lead LI. Conversely, a bundle situated in the right heart is likely to give a negative delta wave in leads V1–V3 and a positive delta wave in lead LI. Sometimes the conduction via the accessory pathway may be intermittent and the ECG may look entirely normal. The ECG also looks normal if there is a retrograde conducting accessory pathway.

The differential diagnosis of WPW syndrome is important. In type A syndrome, the dominant R wave can be mistaken for RVH, RBBB, or a true posterior wall MI. In type B WPW syndrome, the negative delta wave in lead V1 may be mistaken for a LBBB pattern. In WPW syndrome the presence of Q waves or QS waves in any of the leads do not represent a MI. WPW syndrome is found in 1–3/1000 of the population but less than a quarter are accompanied by tachycardia.

2 The common arrhythmias associated with WPW syndrome are AV re-entrant tachycardia (AVRT) or pre-excited AF associated with a risk of progressing to ventricular fibrillation. AV nodal blocking drugs do not slow conduction in the bundle of Kent and are therefore of no use. Digoxin may paradoxically increase conduction down the accessory pathway and increase the ventricular rate. The best way to terminate the tachyarrhythmia is DC cardioversion. Drugs that slow conduction in the accessory pathway such as disopyramide, flecainide, or amiodarone can also be used.

3 ECG 14b shows sinus rhythm, a short PR interval, and a negative delta wave in lead V1 (arrows) characteristic of WPW type B syndrome. There are also delta waves visible in leads L1, V4–V6 (arrows).

4 WPW syndrome may be associated with mitral valve prolapse or Ebstein's anomaly.

14a

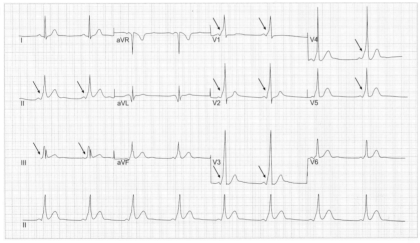

14b

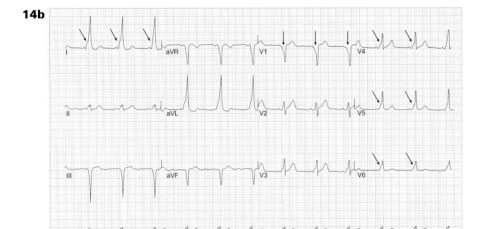

Question 15

A 65-year-old male presented with a history of light-headedness. **ECG 15a** was taken. Five days later, **ECG 15b** was taken in the accident and emergency department after he had a blackout with loss of consciousness lasting for about 1 minute.

1 What are the findings in **ECG 15a**?
2 What are the findings in **ECG 15b**?
3 How should this patient be managed?

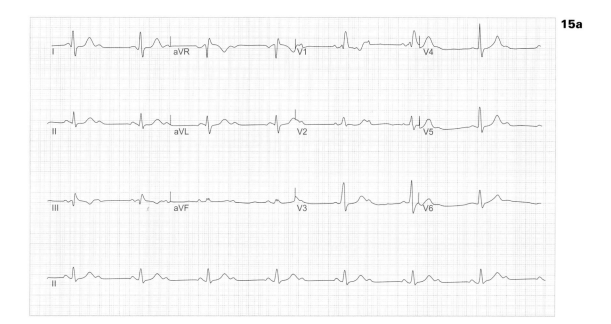

15a

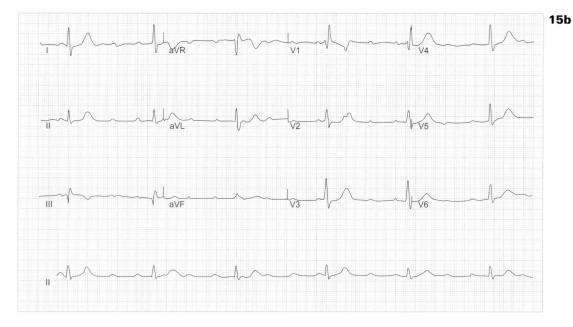

15b

Answer 15

1 ECG 15a shows bradycardia (43 bpm) in the presence of a 2:1 Mobitz type II heart block. There are two P waves (arrows) for every QRS complex. There is a constant PR interval in the conducted beats. The QRS complex shows the presence of a RBBB pattern (circle). First degree and Mobitz type I (Wenckebach) heart blocks may not have serious consequences and may be found in athletes who have a high vagal tone. However, Mobitz type II heart blocks are usually associated with organic heart disease and a significant number of these patients may proceed to develop a complete heart block. In Mobitz type II, the block is usually distal to the AV node.

2 ECG 15b shows complete heart block. There is complete AV dissociation, with the P waves having no relation to the QRS complexes and the PR interval being different in every beat (arrows).

3 This patient requires a permanent pacemaker.

15a

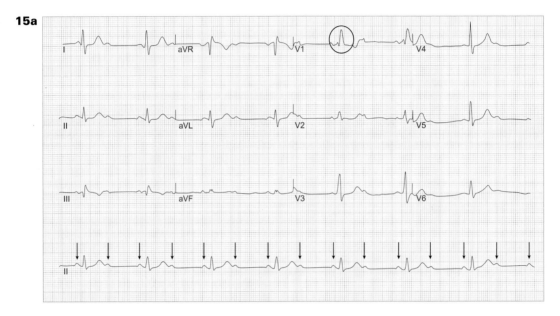

15b

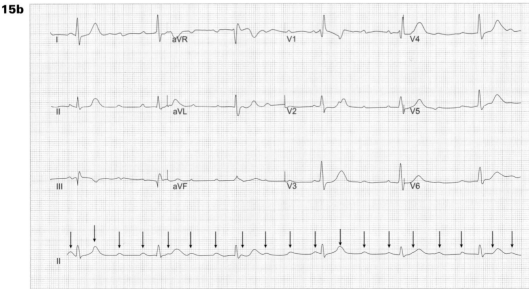

Question 16

A 57-year-old male walked into the accident and emergency department complaining of light-headedness and palpitations. He had a past history of intermittent palpitations. His BP was 130/70 mmHg (17.3/9.3 kPa) and his chest was clear. His CXR showed cardiomegaly but clear lung fields. **ECG 16a** (recorded at 2.5 mm/mV) was taken on admission.

1 What is the differential diagnosis and how should this patient be managed?
2 **ECG 16b** was taken shortly after treatment. What are the findings and what is the final diagnosis?

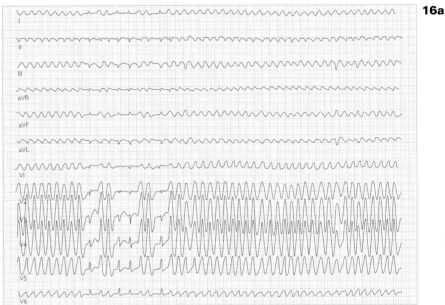

16a

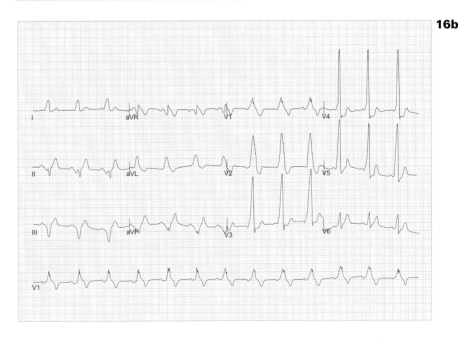

16b

Answer 16

1 ECG 16a shows a broad complex tachycardia with an irregularly irregular rapid ventricular rate. The differential diagnosis includes AF with aberrant conduction and ventricular tachycardia (VT). This is a difficult ECG to interpret, with features that might suggest both supraventricular and ventricular origins. The irregularly irregular rhythm points towards AF. In the chest leads one can notice a ventricular concordance with a number of normally conducted QRS complexes (arrows) that might be considered to be capture beats, suggesting a ventricular origin. In view of the uncertainty of diagnosis electrical cardioversion was performed following which the patient reverted to sinus rhythm.

2 ECG 16b shows sinus rhythm with a short PR interval and a delta wave in the chest leads (arrows) confirming the diagnosis of WPW syndrome. Upright R waves in leads V1 and V2 suggest type A WPW syndrome.

The features against a diagnosis of VT are that the patient was haemodynamically stable and the rhythm was totally irregular. There were also no predisposing factors to develop VT such as ischaemic heart disease or cardiomyopathy. The most likely rhythm on admission, therefore, was AF on the background of WPW syndrome.

16a

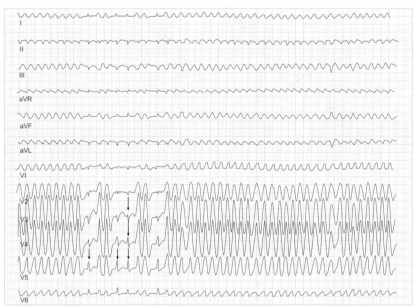

16b

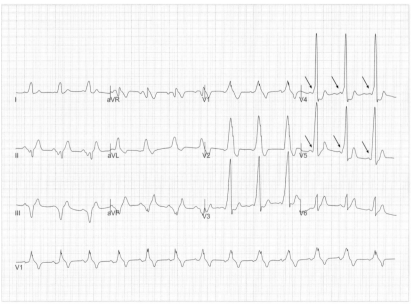

Question 17

ECG 17a was found in an asymptomatic 77-year-old male.

> 1 What are the findings in **ECG 17a**?
> 2 **ECG 17b** is from another patient. What does it show?
> 3 What is the significance of these changes in both ECGs?

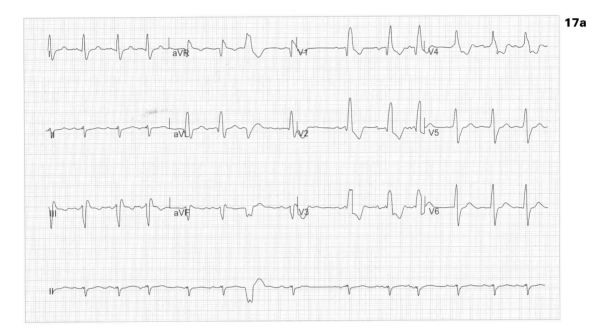

17a

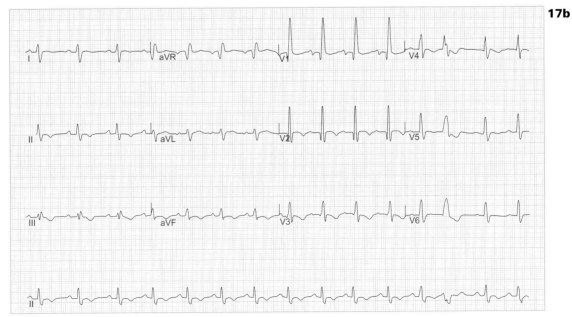

17b

Answer 17

1 ECG 17a shows sinus rhythm with a marked left axis deviation (LAD) (-60°) due to a left anterior hemiblock together with a complete RBBB (rSR pattern in leads V1 and V2 [circles]). This combination is referred to as a bifascicular block. A ventricular ectopic (arrows) can be seen demonstrating a bizarre QRS morphology.

2 ECG 17b shows sinus rhythm with a right axis deviation(RAD) (+100°) suggesting a left posterior hemiblock. There is a complete RBBB. Pathological Q waves are visible in leads V1–V2 (arrows), with T wave inversion seen in leads V1–V5. The ST segments are isoelectric. These changes suggest old anterior wall MI.

Hemiblock is the term used when there is a conduction defect in one of the two main divisions of the left bundle branch. During normal conduction an impulse runs down the anterior and posterior branches of the left bundle simultaneously, activating the anterior and posterior papillary muscles of the left ventricle. When the anterior division is blocked the impulse runs down the posterior branch first, producing an upward movement of the QRS axis and a considerable LAD of ≥-60°. There may be a small Q wave in lead LI and a small R wave in lead LIII. In left anterior hemiblock the QRS duration may be slightly increased by 0.01–0.02 seconds. Conversely, a block in the posterior division of the left bundle (left posterior hemiblock) leads to a RAD of ≥+120°, a small R wave in lead LI, a small Q wave in LIII, and a normal QRS complex. These changes can be seen in right ventricular hypertrophy (RVH) as well. Hence this must be excluded before the diagnosis is made.

3 Both these ECGs are examples of bifascicular blocks. The first ECG is a combination of RBBB and left anterior hemiblock. The second ECG is a combination of RBBB and left posterior hemiblock. Patients with multifascicular blocks are likely to progress to higher degrees of block, eventually requiring a permanent pacemaker. In the second example bifascicular block has occurred in association with an anterior wall MI. This combination represents a poor longer term prognosis.

17a

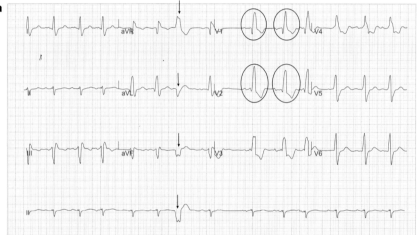

17b

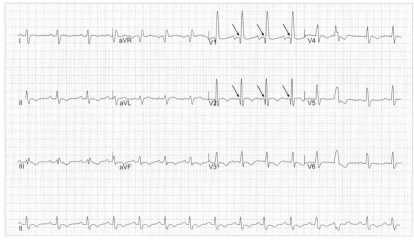

Question 18

A 69-year-old female known to suffer from chronic obstructive airway disease was noted to have an irregularly irregular pulse.

1 What are the findings in **ECG 18**?
2 What is the significance of these findings?

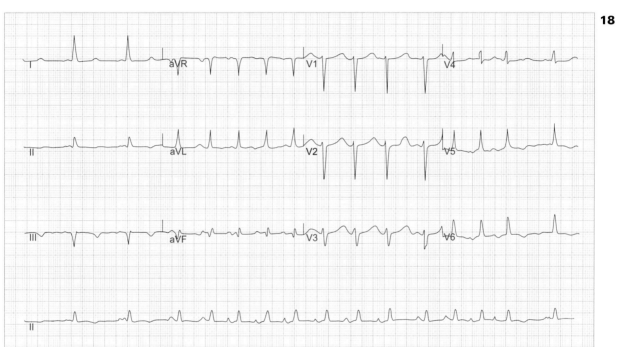

18

Answer 18

1 ECG 18 shows irregular rhythm with QRS complexes preceded by P waves of varying morphology and PR intervals (arrows). This is due to a wandering atrial pacemaker.

2 This is a relatively benign condition that does not require any specific treatment. The initiating focus in this condition includes both the SA node and other ectopic foci in the atria and AV node. Its aetiology is not understood. Clinically it can be easily mistaken for AF. It is therefore, important to perform an electrocardiogram to differentiate between the two conditions because of their different therapeutic and prognostic implications.

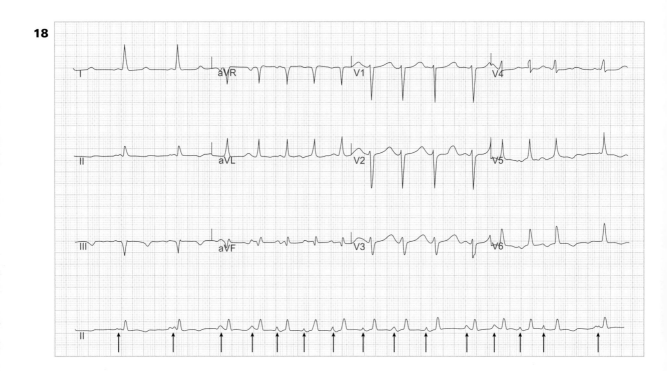

Question 19

A 60-year-old male presented with a history of central crushing chest pain. On examination his BP was 80/60 mmHg (10.7/8.0 kPa) and he had engorged neck veins. His chest was clear.

1 What are the findings in **ECG 19a**?
2 What does the clinical presentation suggest and what does **ECG 19b** show?

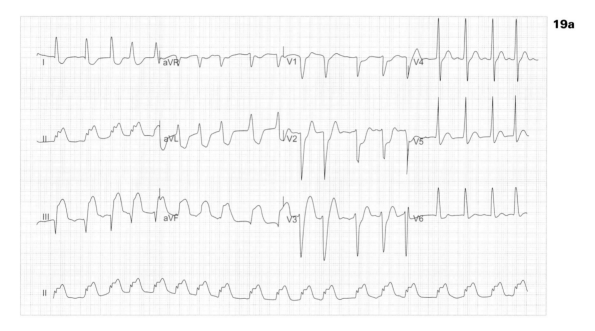

19a

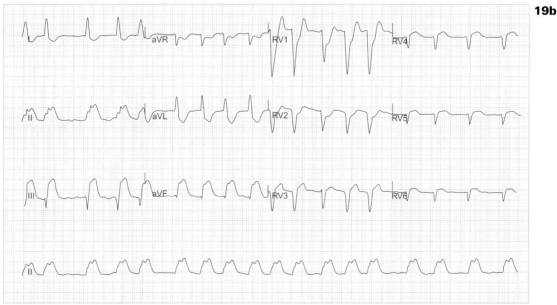

19b

Right precordial leads

Answer 19

1 ECG 19a shows AF and changes consistent with acute inferior wall MI, showing typical ST segment elevation in leads LII, LIII, and aVF, and reciprocal ST segment changes in leads VI and V2. There is marked ST segment depression in leads LI and aVL indicating lateral wall ischaemia.

2 The clinical presentation of this patient with hypotension, engorged neck veins, and ST elevation in the inferior leads strongly points to a diagnosis of right ventricular infarction. Right-sided precordial leads are important in establishing the diagnosis. ST segment elevation of ≥1 mm in lead RV4 (circles) confirms the diagnosis, as seen in **ECG 19b**. This may be a transient change. The ECG should therefore be performed early. Other changes are ST segment elevation, greater in lead LIII as compared with lead LII. This difference should be ≥1 mm.

Transthoracic echocardiography carried out in the acute stage can be useful in providing a diagnosis by showing a poorly contracting and dilated right ventricle (RV). Isolated RV infarction occurs in less than 3% of all MI. In 50% of all inferior wall infarcts there is associated RV infarction, which is haemodynamically significant in only 5% of cases. The inpatient mortality in haemodynamically significant RV infarction is about 30%.

However, the long-term mortality of patients surviving the acute event is 6%, similar to an uncomplicated inferior wall MI. This high inpatient mortality highlights the importance of early diagnosis and appropriate management. Intravenous fluid replacement is crucial in the management of these patients to maintain high right-sided filling pressures. Diamorphine, intravenous nitrates, diuretics, and inotropic agents such as dobutamine and dopamine can have detrimental effects when given alone without appropriate fluid replacement.

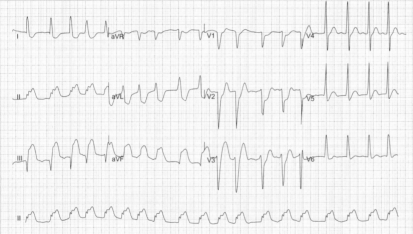

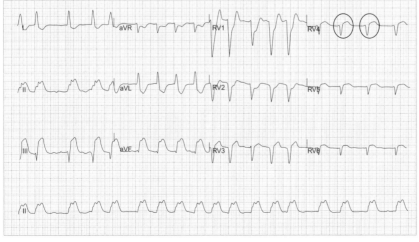

Right precordial leads

Question 20

A 76-year-old retired miner presented with shortness of breath. On clinical examination he was noted to be centrally cyanosed and had prominent 'a' waves on his jugular venous pressure. **ECG 20** was recorded.

> **1** What are the findings in **ECG 20**?
> **2** What is the diagnosis?

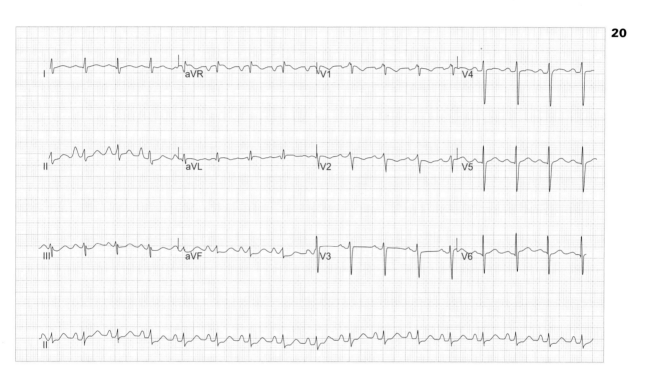

20

Answer 20

1 ECG 20 shows sinus rhythm with prominent peaked P waves in LII, LIII, and aVF (arrows). There is S1 S2 S3 pattern in the limb leads, as well as persistent deep S waves in leads V5 and V6 giving a clockwise rotation (circles).

2 The ECG shows evidence of cor pulmonale. Criteria for right atrial hypertrophy is a P wave that is ≥2.5 mm in height in leads LII, LIII, aVF, or V2. The characteristic findings in cor pulmonale include tall peaked P waves (P pulmonale), RAD, and clockwise rotation. In severe cases of pulmonary hypertension, RVH may develop. Criteria for RVH include an R wave in lead V1 of ≥7mm, an R wave in lead V1 plus an S wave in leads V5 or V6 of ≥10mm, a deeper S than R wave in lead V6, and a taller R than S wave in lead V1. There may be other associated features that include a RAD of ≥90°, a strain pattern in leads V1 and V2, RBBB, S1 S2 S3 pattern, and a clockwise rotation. P pulmonale waves may also be seen in massive pulmonary embolism, pulmonary stenosis, tricuspid stenosis, and tricuspid incompetence.

20

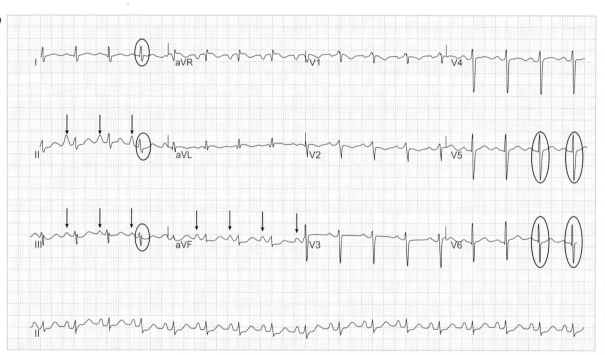

Question 21

A 58-year-old female with no previous history of ischaemic heart disease presented with palpitations. **ECG 21** was taken in the accident and emergency department.

1 What are the findings in **ECG 21**?
2 What is their significance?

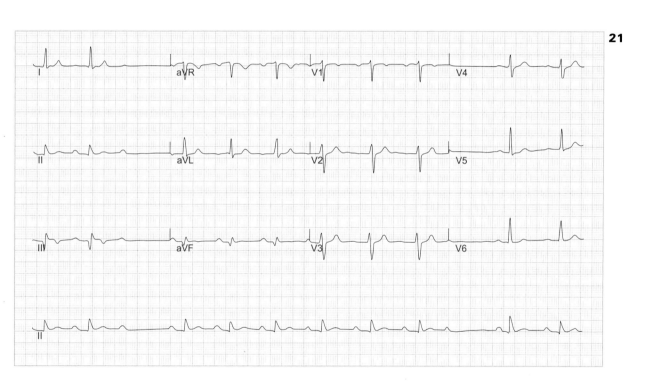

21

Answer 21

1 ECG 21 shows a Wenckebach phenomenon also known as Mobitz type I heart block. The changes are best observed in the rhythm strip at the bottom of the ECG. There is progressive prolongation of the PR interval followed by dropped QRS complexes (arrows).

2 Mobitz type I heart block may be a physiological finding but is most commonly associated with the occlusion of the right coronary artery leading to ischaemia of the AV node. It does not appear to affect survival. It occurs in 4–10% of patients with acute inferior wall MI and is usually transient and does not persist for >72 hours after infarction. It may be intermittent and rarely progresses to complete heart block. It occurs due to a gradual increase in the relative refractory period of the tissue, which becomes increasingly impaired until it finally fails completely and a beat is dropped.

21

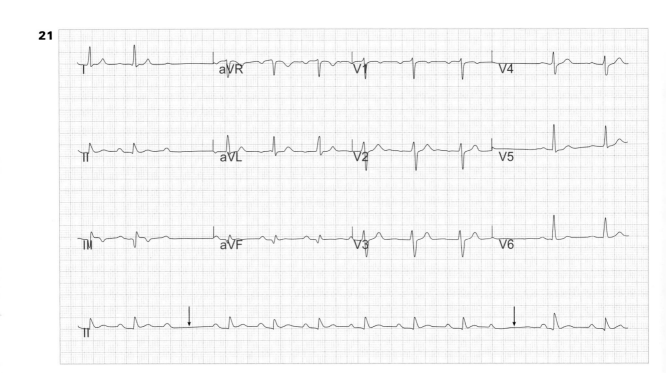

22 Question 22

A 78-year-old male presented with palpitations and shortness of breath.

1 **ECG 22a** was taken shortly after admission. What are the findings in this ECG?
2 **ECG 22b** was taken from another patient found collapsed. What does it show?

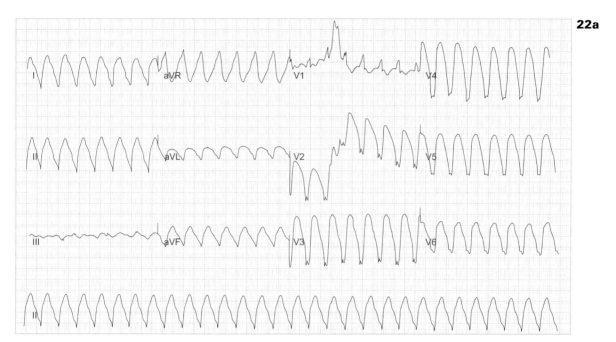

22a

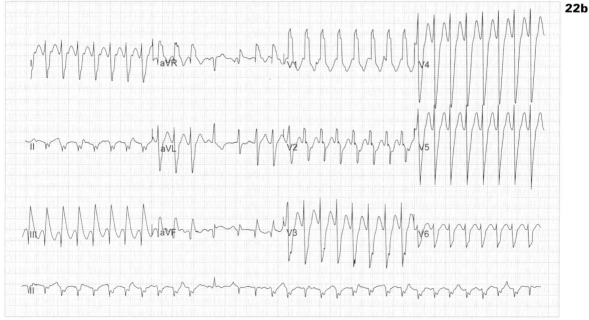

22b

Answer 22

1 ECG 22a shows a broad complex tachycardia with a rate of 175 bpm. There are a number of features that favour a VT rather than an SVT with aberrant conduction. The QRS complexes are wide (>140 ms) and demonstrate a marked axis deviation. There is concordance with the QRS complexes all pointing in the same direction. There is evidence of atrial activity and P waves (arrows) can be seen distorting QRS complexes but with no set pattern, indicating AV dissociation.

2 ECG 22b is another example of a VT showing a number of other additional features that point towards the diagnosis. There is evidence of P wave activity dissociated from the QRS complexes (V1 [arrows]). In lead aVL there is a fusion beat (circle 1) followed by a capture beat (circle 2). Fusion beats occur when an atrial beat 'makes it through' to the ventricles and causes simultaneous depolarization at the same time as the ventricular impulse. One can see a P wave followed by a QRS complex with a normal morphology in its initial phase, but with characteristics of a ventricular ectopic in the later phase. A capture beat is a normally conducted sinus beat that is captured by the ventricles. Its morphology is like a normal P-QRS complex. In SVT the ECG pattern is usually RBBB while in VT it may be either RBBB or LBBB. In VT, as in this case, the RBBB demonstrates an Rsr shape with the tip of the S wave well above the isoelectric line in V1 and an RS ratio of <1 in V6. In SVT it has an rSR configuration with the tip of the S wave reaching the isoelectric line in lead V1 and an RS ratio of >1 in lead V6. When there is doubt it is always safer to treat the arrhythmia as VT rather than as SVT.

22a

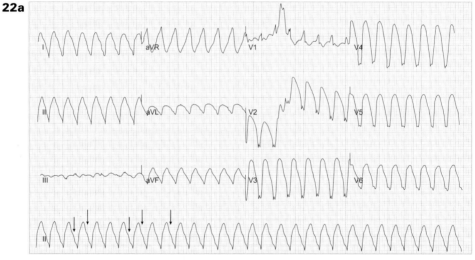

22b

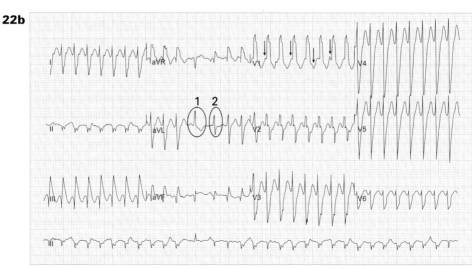

Question 23

An asymptomatic middle-aged male had an electrocardiogram as part of a routine check-up.

What are the findings in **ECG 23**?

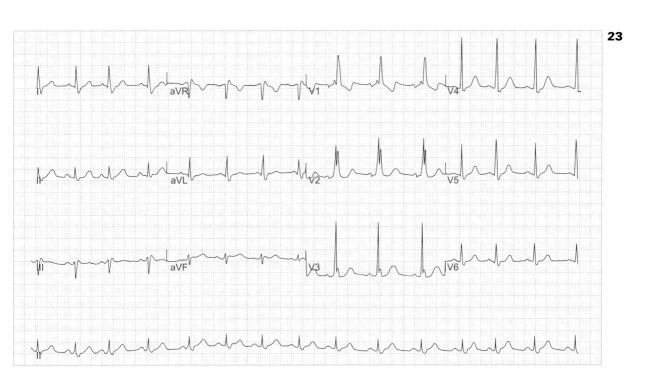

23

Answer 23

ECG 23 shows sinus rhythm and typical features of complete RBBB. The duration of the QRS complex is >0.12 seconds. There is an rSR pattern with a secondary R wave in leads V1 (circles) and a deep S wave with a slurred upslope in the lateral leads LI, aVL, and V6 (arrows).

RBBB may be an incidental finding. However, it can be a manifestation of a variety of cardiac disorders including ischaemic heart disease, pulmonary embolism, pulmonary hypertension, cor pulmonale, cardiomyopathy, and hypertension. When conduction is blocked down the right bundle, the electrical impulse flows down the left branch activating the left ventricle, after which it passes through the interventricular septum from left to right to activate the right ventricle.

This is a normal sequence of conduction but with delayed activation of the right ventricle. Because of this sequence of depolarization the BBB has no effect on the initial part of the QRS complex. The main features of RBBB are: a broad QRS complex reflecting delayed ventricular depolarization, an M-shaped rSR complex in leads V1 and V2, and slurred and widened S waves in leads V5–V6 and leads LI and aVL. The ST segment and T wave are opposite to the terminal QRS. As the initial part of the QRS complex is not affected in MI, a pathological Q wave can be seen even if superimposed on a RBBB.

23

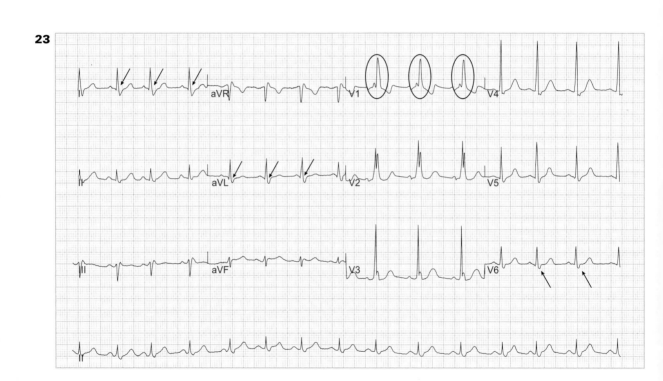

Question 24

A 71-year-old male presented with a history of dizzy spells. On examination he was noted to have a systolic murmur.

1 What are the findings in **ECG 24**?
2 How do these abnormalities correlate with the patient's symptoms?

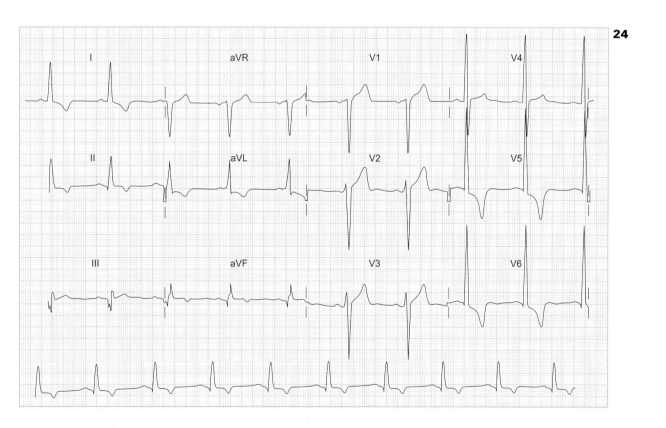

24

Answer 24

1 ECG 24 shows normal sinus rhythm and normal axis. There are tall R waves in leads V4–V6, LI, and aVL. There are deep S waves in leads V1 and V2. There is deep T wave inversion in leads LI, LII, aVL, aVF, and V5–V6. The ECG shows the voltage criteria for LVH, with a strain pattern.

LVH is suspected if: R waves in any one or more of leads V5–V6 are taller than 25 mm, or the sum of the tallest R wave in lead V5 and the deepest S wave in lead V2 is ≥35 mm, or the S wave in one or more of leads V1–V2 exceeds 25 mm, or the R wave in lead aVL exceeds 13 mm. These criteria are strongly suggestive but not diagnostic, as these changes may also be found in young, thin people with normal hearts. One must also look for evidence of a strain pattern, seen by ST segment depression and T wave inversion (arrows) in anterolateral leads, as it strongly suggests the diagnosis of LVH.

2 The changes in the ECG are suggestive of LVH. The presence of a systolic murmur suggests the possibility of aortic stenosis or, less likely, a hypertrophic cardiomyopathy. The diagnosis should be confirmed by echocardiography. Long-standing hypertension is the commonest cause of LVH.

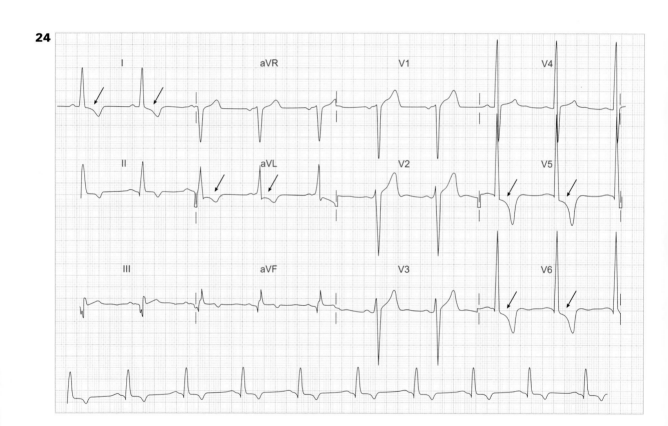

Question 25

A 41-year-old female who had a history of heavy smoking presented with central crushing chest pain of 1 hour duration.

1 What are the findings in **ECG 25**?
2 What is the prognosis of this condition?

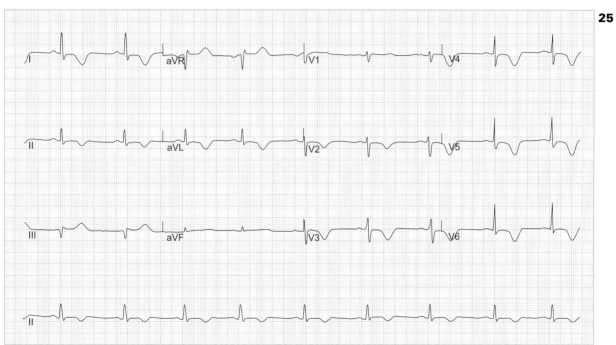

25

Answer 25

1 ECG 25 shows sinus rhythm and normal axis. There is symmetrical T wave inversion in leads LI, aVL, and V2–V6 (arrows). These changes are suggestive of non-ST elevation MI (NSTEMI). It is also known as a non-Q wave or subendocardial infarction or, more appropriately, partial thickness MI. The diagnosis is confirmed by elevation of cardiac enzymes such as CK/CKMB, ALT, LDH, and other cardiac markers such as cardiac troponins (troponin T and troponin I). The term subendocardial infarction is a misnomer since this is, in fact, a partial thickness infarction.

2 It is important to follow up these patients since the prognosis is usually worse compared with that for transmural infarction. Although they have a lower inpatient mortality compared to patients with transmural infarcts (2.0% versus 12–18%), their late mortality (1 year) rate is high. They also have a higher incidence of post infarct angina and arrhythmias compared with that for transmural infarcts. Patients who sustain sub-endocardial MI still have viable myocardium, which is at higher risk of sustaining further damage. These patients may therefore benefit from early investigation and re-vascularization to improve the prognosis.

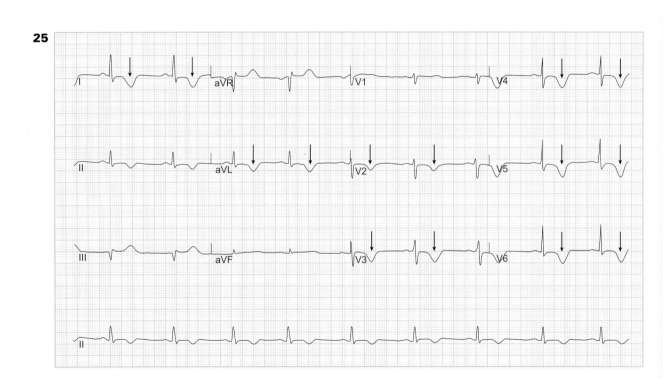

25

Question 26

A 72-year-old male had symptoms of dizzy spells and blackouts. He was found to be in complete heart block and had a permanent pacemaker implanted. After a temporary improvement he developed the symptoms again.

1 What are the findings in **ECG 26**?
2 What further investigations should be considered?

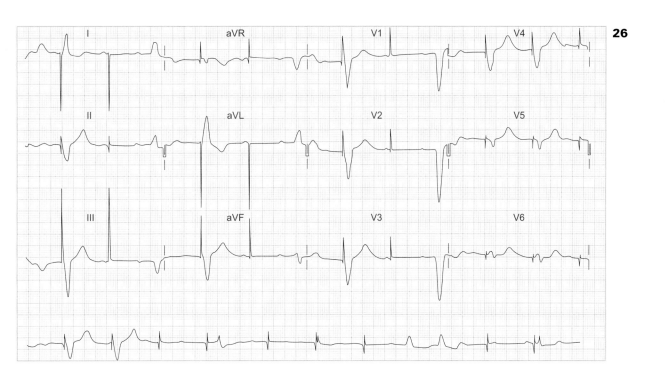

26

Answer 26

1 ECG 26 shows a failed single chamber pacemaker. Ventricular pacing spikes can be seen occurring at regular intervals. On the rhythm strip ventricular capture beats can be seen in the first two complexes (circles), followed by persistent failure of ventricular capture in all subsequent beats (arrows). Here the QRS complexes are seen to occur independent of the pacing spikes.
2 A CXR and a pacemaker check should be requested. In this patient the CXR revealed the displacement of the ventricular lead from its original position. After repositioning the lead, the patient became symptom free.

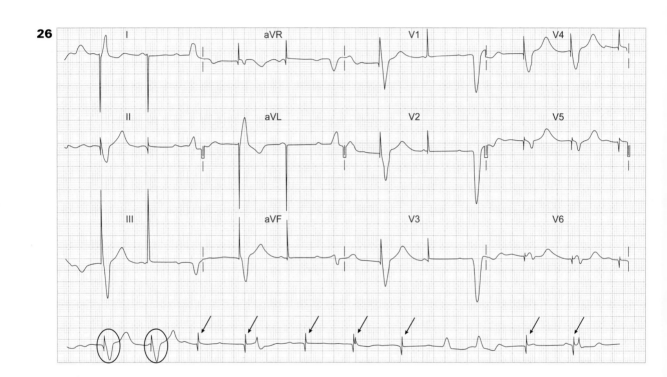

Question 27

A 42-year-old female developed palpitations and progressive shortness of breath. Her symptoms were preceded by an upper respiratory tract infection 2 weeks ago. A CXR revealed cardiomegaly.

What are the findings in **ECG 27**?

27

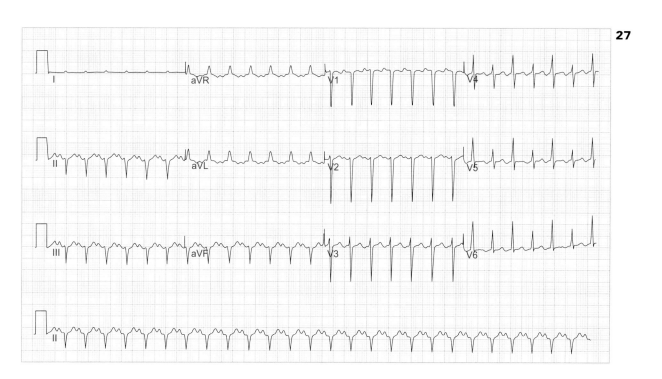

Answer 27

ECG 27 shows sinus tachycardia at a rate of 163 bpm. The QRS complexes in leads LI, aVR, and aVL are of low voltage. Each QRS complex is preceded by a P wave of normal morphology. The PR interval is normal. There is variation in the height of the QRS complexes best seen in leads V3–V6 (arrows). This shows electrical alternans.

Electrical alternans occurs when the height (voltage) of the QRS complexes varies. It is often found in association with a pericardial effusion leading to tamponade. In this lady it was confirmed on transthoracic echocardiography.

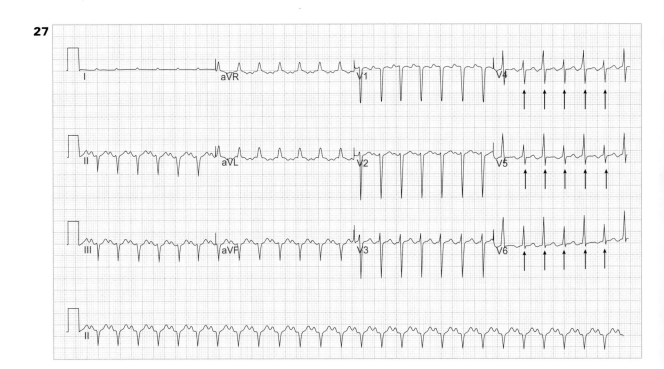

Question 28

A 25-year-old male with a history of palpitations was found to have **ECG 28**.

What are the findings in **ECG 28**?

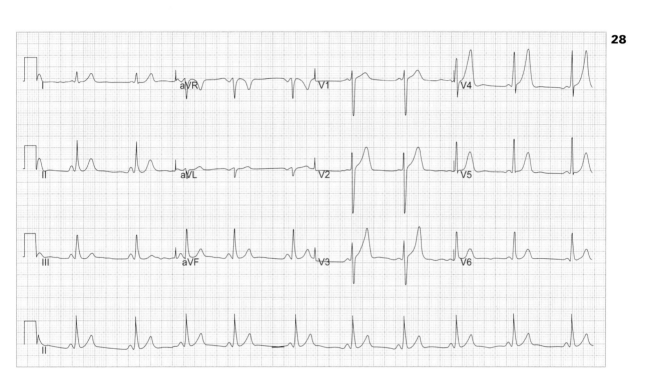

28

Answer 28

ECG 28 shows sinus rhythm with a normal axis. The P waves are normal but there is a short PR interval of 0.10 seconds (arrows). The QRS complexes are normal and there are no ST segment abnormalities. The ECG and history are suggestive of the Lown–Ganong–Levine (LGL) syndrome. It is the result of an aberrant AV pathway and is characterized by a short PR interval of ≤0.12 seconds, normal QRS complexes, and the absence of a delta wave. It may lead to attacks of atrial tachycardia.

28

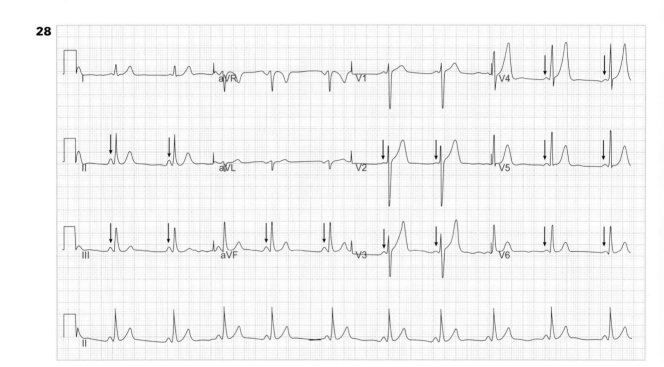

Question 29

A 61-year-old diabetic male was admitted after being involved in a serious road traffic accident. He had a past history of angina. **ECG 29** was taken on admission.

> 1 What are the findings in **ECG 29**?
> 2 Should this patient be thrombolysed?
> 3 What further investigation is required?

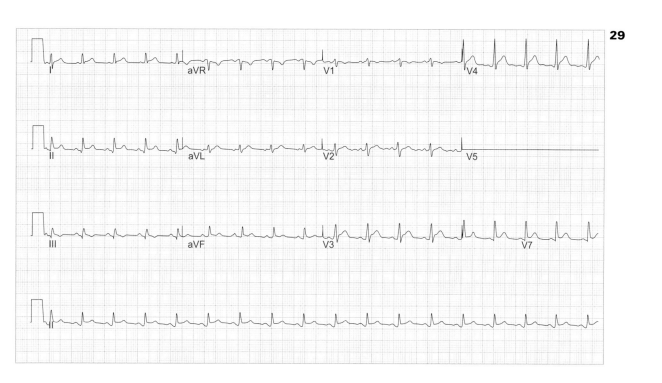

29

Answer 29

1 ECG 29 shows sinus rhythm with normal P waves, PR interval, and QRS complexes. The Q wave in leads II and III are nonpathological. There is an ST segment elevation seen both in the inferior leads LII, aVF and in the anterior leads V3, V4, and V7 (arrows). Leads V5 and V6 are missing because of a dressing on the chest wall.

2 This patient should not be thrombolysed. Severe trauma is a relative contraindication to thrombolysis. Despite the past history of angina and risk factor status of the patient, these changes are consistent with myocardial contusion. A clue to this can be seen from the ECG where lead V5 and V6 could not be positioned.

   Cardiac damage may be caused by penetrating and nonpenetrating injury to the chest. Serious cardiac damage can occur even in the absence of visible external trauma. Any cardiac structure may be involved. Myocardial contusion may cause arrhythmias, BBB patterns, and changes resembling those of an acute MI. Impaired left ventricular function may be noted. Pericardial effusions may complicate serious trauma and can develop up to several weeks after the incident. Trauma to the heart can also result in rupture of valves, atrial or ventricular walls, and of major vessels.

3 Echocardiography is required as it may confirm myocardial contusion, any valve injury, ruptured vessels, or significant pericardial effusion including cardiac tamponade.

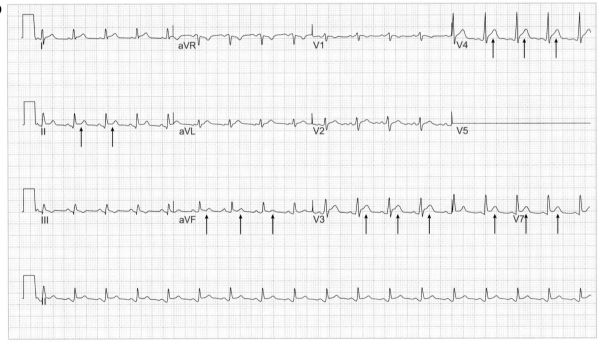

Question 30

A 59-year-old male had symptoms of palpitations and dizzy spells. Twenty-four hour Holter monitoring revealed evidence of sick sinus syndrome and paroxysmal AF. It also revealed sinus arrest with pauses of up to 3.2 seconds. He was on no medical treatment and required a permanent pacemaker.

1 What are the findings in **ECG 30**?
2 What nomenclature is used to describe methods of pacing?
3 What type of pacemaker has been used and how can it help in paroxysmal AF associated with sick sinus syndrome?

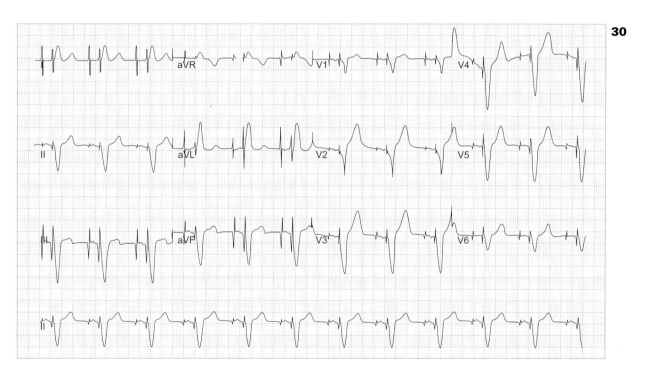

30

Answer 30

1 ECG 30 shows the presence of a dual chamber (DDD) pacemaker as evidenced by two pacing spikes. The first spike (circle) is followed by a P wave and the second spike (arrow) is followed by a broad QRS complex, confirming its ventricular origin.

2 A three letters code (*Table*, below) is used to describe methods of pacing. The majority of modern pacemakers are VVI or DDD. VVO pacemakers that pace ventricles at a fixed rate without sensing are not used any more, due to the risk of precipitating ventricular arrhythmias.

3 A dual chamber (DDD) pacemaker can help to re-establish and maintain sinus rhythm in sick sinus syndrome, by restoring the normal atrioventricular relationship by sequential pacing of the atria and ventricles. In sick sinus syndrome, AF is usually pause dependent. It arises from multiple atrial foci discharging simultaneously during periods of sinus arrest. Sinus rhythm can be maintained by maintaining atrioventricular synchrony.

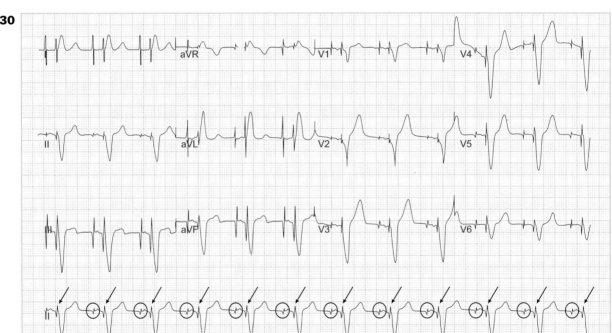

Pacemaker coding

First letter	Second letter	Third letter
Chamber paced	Chamber sensed	Response to sensing
A atrial pacing	O no sensing	O no response
V ventricular pacing	A atrial sensing	I inhibited
D dual chamber pacing	V ventricular sensing	T triggered
	D dual chamber sensing	D pulse triggering and inhibition

Question 31

An 80-year-old female was having blackouts. During carotid sinus massage (CSM) she developed dizziness and light-headedness. **ECG 31** was taken.

1 What is the diagnosis?
2 How should this condition be treated?

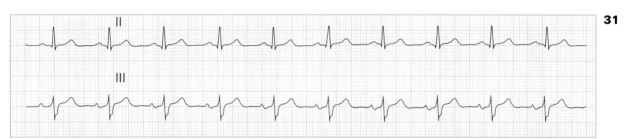

Before carotid sinus massage

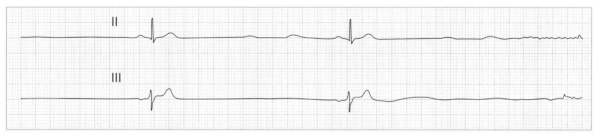

During carotid sinus massage

Answer 31

1 The history and ECG in this lady suggest the diagnosis of carotid sinus syndrome (CSS). **ECG 31** shows a significant pause of >3 seconds on CSM. When such a pause is present in association with symptoms, the diagnosis is CSS. If the pause is present without any symptoms, the diagnosis is carotid sinus hypersensitivity (CSH). There are three subtypes of CSS: (1) cardioinhibitory, when CSM results in a pause of ≥3 seconds with symptoms; (2) vasodepressor, when CSM results in a drop in systolic blood pressure of ≥50 mmHg (6.7 kPa) with symptoms; and (3) mixed, when both the above criteria are present.

2 Drugs that depress the SA or AV node should be stopped. According to the ACC/AHA guidelines, recurrent syncope related to pauses of ≥3 seconds during CSM in the absence of drugs is an indication for a permanent pacemaker. The indication for a permanent pacemaker is not so clear when the bradycardia is not closely related to symptoms. A dual chamber pacemaker (DDD/DVI) is preferred in this situation.

The vasodepressor component of CSS is more difficult to treat. Vasodilator medication should be stopped. Selective serotonin re-uptake inhibitors or beta blockers have been used to try to improve the symptoms in patients with CSS.

31

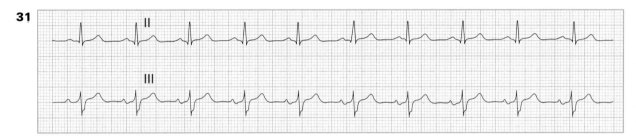

Before carotid sinus massage

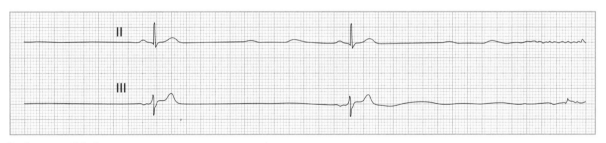

During carotid sinus massage

Question 32

A 58-year-old male presented in the accident and emergency department with chest pain.

1 What are the findings in **ECG 32a**?
2 What does **ECG 32b** show?
3 What is the differential diagnosis of a tall R wave in V1?

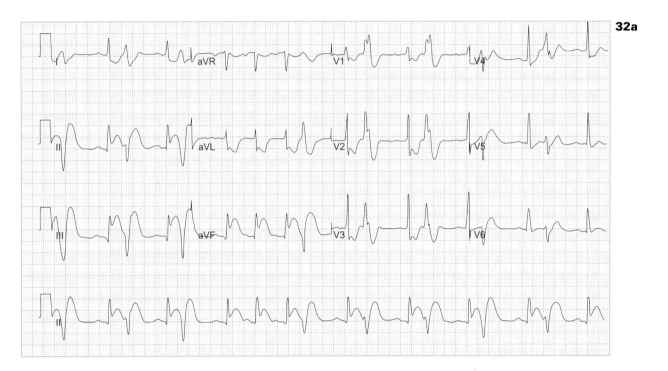
32a

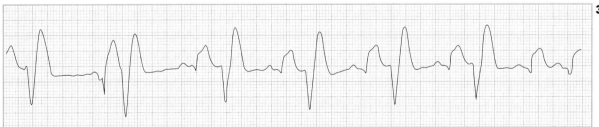
32b

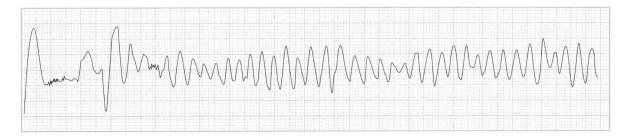

Answer 32

1 ECG 32a shows ST segment elevation in leads LII, LIII, and aVF consistent with acute inferior wall MI (arrows). There is a tall R wave in lead V1 and V2 (circles) indicating posterior wall extension. There are frequent ventricular ectopics some of which are falling on the T waves of the preceding QRS complexes (arrows in rhythm strip). This is known as 'R on T' phenomenon. This can lead to dangerous ventricular tachyarrhythmias.

2 ECG 32b is the rhythm strip from the same patient. There are frequent ventricular ectopics shown in this rhythm strip, one of which is an 'R on T' (arrow). In the second part of the rhythm strip there is ventricular fibrillation precipitated after such an event (circle).

3 ECG 32a shows an example of a tall R wave in V1. The differential diagnosis is posterior wall infarction, RBBB, acute pulmonary embolism, RVH, WPW type A, and a normal variant in the newborn.

32a

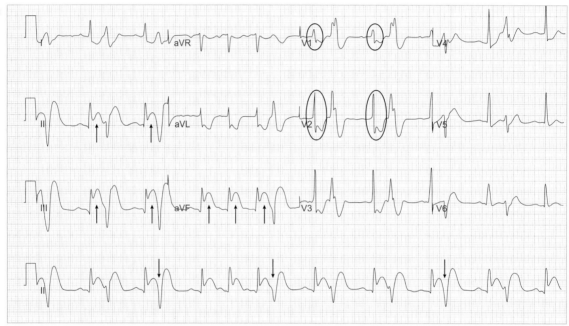

32b

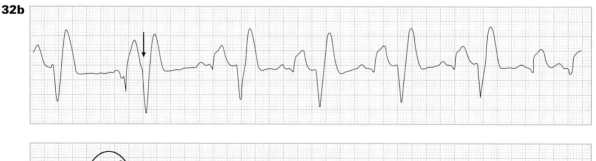

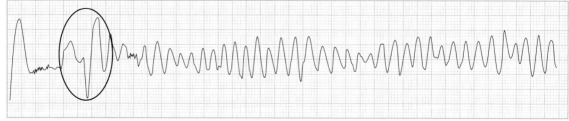

Question 33

A 75-year-old female with a past history of ischaemic heart disease presented with chest pain of 45 minutes duration. She had an ECG performed in the accident and emergency department.

1 What are the findings in **ECG 33**?
2 Should this patient be thrombolysed?

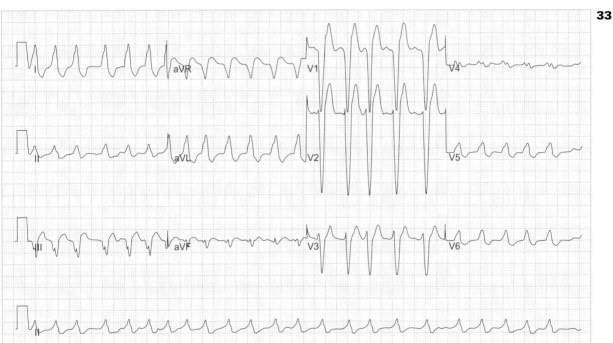

33

Answer 33

1 ECG 33 shows broad complex tachycardia. The RR interval is irregularly irregular. There are no recognizable P waves. The QRS complexes are broad showing a LBBB pattern. The diagnosis is AF with a rapid ventricular rate and LBBB. Some times LBBB may be transient related to a fast heart rate. Other heart blocks such as RBBB and fascicular blocks may also transiently appear with faster rates.

2 In the presence of LBBB the patient should only be thrombolysed when there is a good history of chest pain suggestive of MI and new onset of LBBB. In this paticular patient there is a prior history of underlying ischaemic heart disease; therefore, this ECG needs to be compared to the most recent ECG prior to this episode. If this ECG shows no new change compared to the previous ECG, the patient should not be thrombolysed.

33

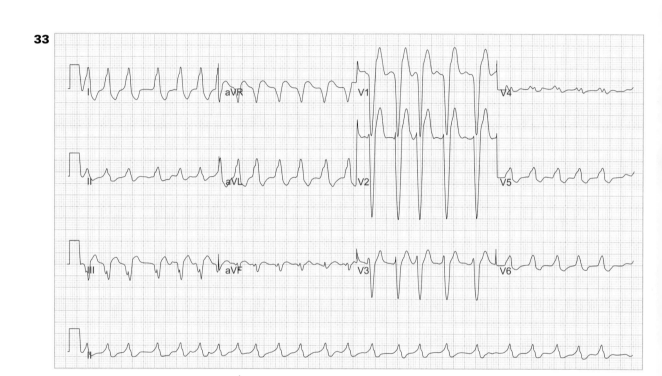

Question 34

A 30-year-old male known to have a heart murmur since childhood, presented with shortness of breath. On examination he was cyanosed and had finger clubbing. **ECG 34** was taken on admission.

What are the findings in **ECG 34**?

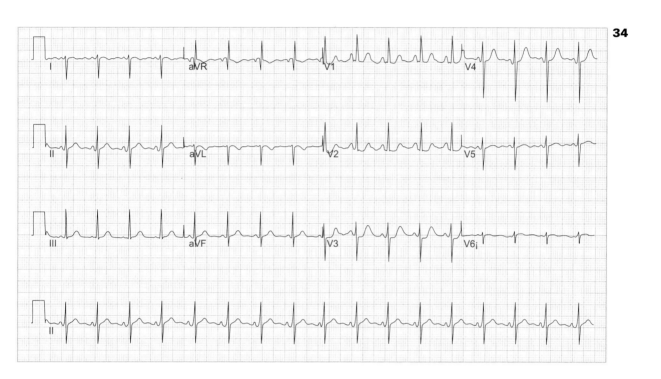

34

Answer 34

ECG 34 shows sinus rhythm with marked RAD (123°). It fulfils several of the criteria of RVH. There is a prominent R wave of >7 mm in lead V1 (arrows). The R waves are taller than the S waves in leads V1 and V2 and there is a deeper S wave than R wave in leads V5 and V6 (arrows). The sum of the R wave in V1 and the S wave in lead V5 is >10 mm.

The clinical presentation in this ECG suggests the presence of a congenital heart defect with pulmonary hypertension and a right to left shunt. This patient had a ventricular septal defect (VSD). An electrocardiogram with a small, uncomplicated VSD may be normal. When a large defect is present, left atrial and left ventricular enlargement occur. LVH, usually with diastolic volume overload pattern, is present in uncomplicated large VSDs. The presence of RAD or the progressive right shift of the QRS axis in the frontal plane suggests RVH secondary to development of pulmonary hypertension. The presence of cyanosis and clubbing and the ECG features suggest the diagnosis of Eisenmenger's syndrome.

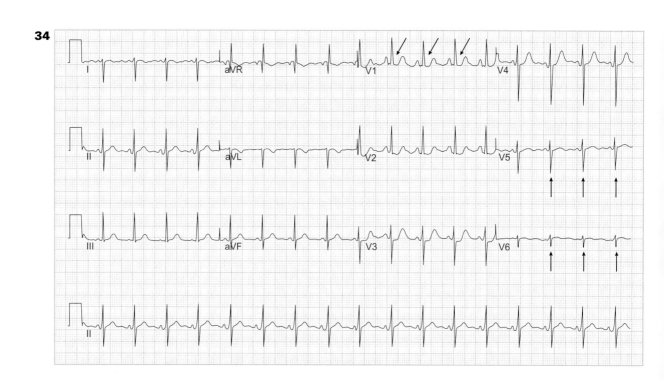

Question 35

A 79-year-old male presented with dizzy spells. **ECG 35a** was taken on admission. He was haemodynamically stable and had normal U&E.

1 What are the findings in **ECG 35a**?
2 What further investigation should be requested?
3 **ECG 35b** is from another patient; what does it show?

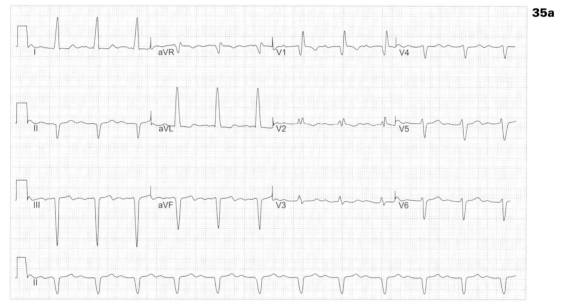
35a

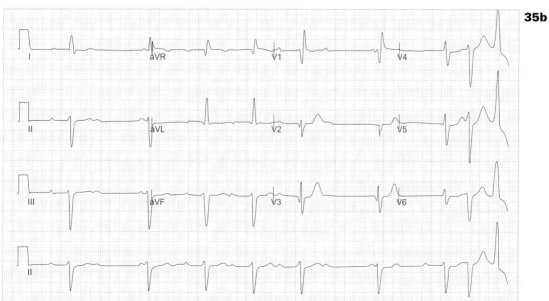
35b

Answer 35

1 ECG 35a shows sinus rhythm. The PR interval is markedly prolonged (324 ms) indicating a first degree heart block (markers). There is LAD due to a left anterior hemiblock. The QRS complexes are broad with an rSR pattern in lead V2 (circles) confirming the presence of RBBB. The ECG shows a trifascicular block. Trifascicular block refers to the presence of first degree heart block, RBBB, together with an incomplete block affecting at least one of the anterior or posterior branches of the left bundle branch. The block has to be partial otherwise the ECG would show complete heart block. Progression to complete heart block may occur.
2 Twenty-four-hour ECG (Holter monitoring) should be requested to rule out intermittent complete heart block leading to Stoke Adam's attacks.
3 ECG 35b shows a Mobitz type I (Wenckebach) heart block. In the rhythm strip one can see a dropped QRS complex (arrow) after the fifth P wave. The PR interval lengthens progressively from P waves 1–5, characteristic of Mobitz type I block. There is LAD due to left anterior hemiblock and RBBB. This is another example of a higher degree of trifascicular block. Such a patient has a higher risk of progression to complete heart block.

35a

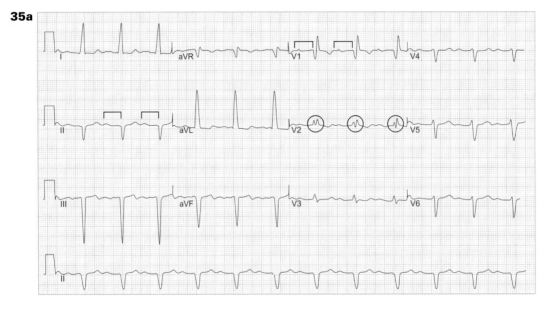

35b

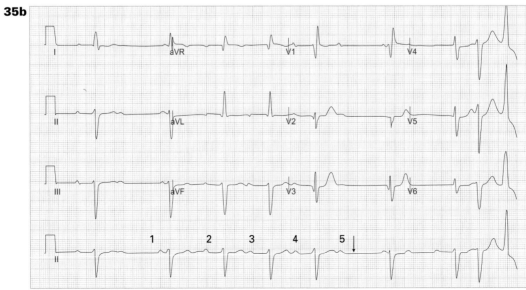

Question 36

A 77-year-old male presented in the accident and emergency department after being found collapsed by his wife. His BP was 110/65 mmHg (14.7/8.7 kPa) and he had a pulse rate of 60 bpm. He was on no medication. An ECG on admission showed evidence of acute inferior wall MI. He was thrombolysed with streptokinase and later developed complete heart block. He required a permanent pacemaker.

1 What are the findings in **ECG 36a**?
2 What type of pacemaker has been used and how can you distinguish between a ventricular single chamber and a dual chamber pacemaker on the ECG?
3 **ECG 36b** is from another patient. What does the rhythm strip show?

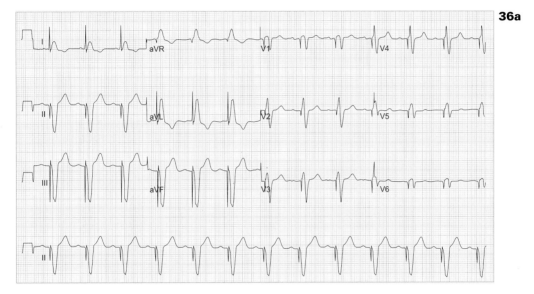

36a

36b

Answer 36

1 ECG 36a shows normal P waves arising from the sinus node followed by a ventricular pacing spike (arrows) and a QRS complex.

2 This patient has a dual chamber (DDD) pacemaker. The clue that this is a DDD pacemaker is that there is atrioventricular synchrony even though there is a history of complete heart block. The purpose of the atrial lead is to sense atrial activity and to pace the atrium if required. This is in contrast to **ECG 30**, where the patient had sick sinus syndrome and because of sinus node disease the atrial lead was pacing as well as sensing. The ventricular lead is generating a pacing spike followed by a QRS complex after atrial sensing. This feature maintains normal physiological delay and AV synchrony.

3 ECG 36b is another example of DDD pacing. The rhythm strip shows adequate sinus rate. Hence the atrial lead senses but does not pace. However, at the 11th complex (circle) there is a transient slowing of the sinus rate and the preprogrammed pacemaker changes its mode and paces the atrium, followed by the ventricle maintaining AV synchrony.

36a

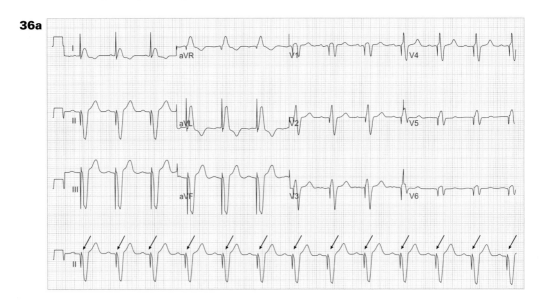

36b

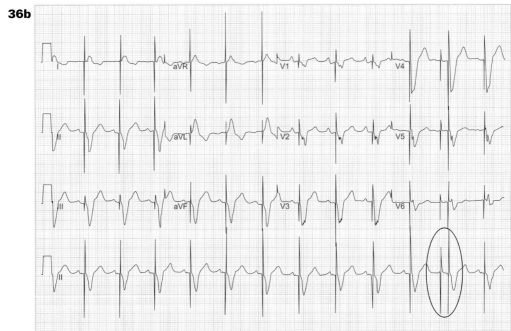

Question 37

A 30-year-old male presented with palpitations, sweating, and light-headedness. He was haemodynamically stable. **ECG 37a** revealed a broad complex tachycardia. He had an electrical cardioversion. **ECG 37b** and **37c** were performed during and just after cardioversion.

1 What are the findings in **ECG 37a**?
2 What complication has developed in **ECG 37b** and why did it occur?
3 How could this complication have been avoided?
4 What does **ECG 37c** show and what is the final diagnosis?

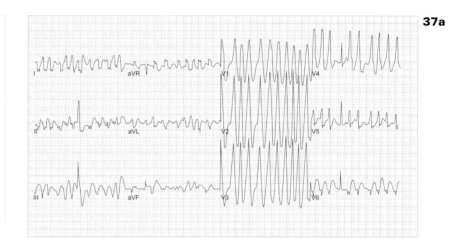

37a

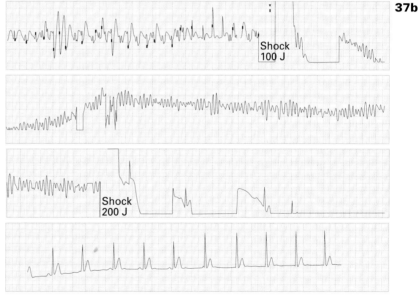

37b

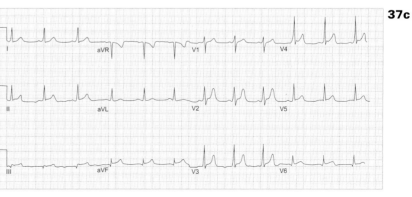

37c

Answer 37

1 ECG 37a shows a broad complex tachycardia with a rate of approximately 210 bpm. The rhythm is irregularly irregular, suggesting rapid AF with aberrant conduction.

2 The rhythm strip in **ECG 37b** demonstrates three different cardiac rhythms. The initial rhythm is rapid AF just prior to cardioversion (A). There are bold vertical markers indicating attempted synchronization of the DC shock. Normally the synchronization should always be on the R wave. The strip however, shows synchronization occurring haphazardly. The last four synchronization markers (arrows) are consistently falling on the T waves, thus resulting in the inappropriate delivery of the DC shock over the T wave. This led to the development of ventricular fibrillation shown in (B). The third rhythm is sinus rhythm (C), which was established after another DC shock of 200 J.

3 To avoid this complication the operator should ensure that synchronization markers are falling on the R wave consistently. Several lead positions on the monitor should be tried and the best lead showing the QRS complexes in the same axis should be chosen. This may be difficult to achieve at times. In such a situation the rhythm should be treated like VT or VF, and higher energy shocks (200 J, 360 J, and 360 J) should be delivered.

4 ECG 37c shows sinus rhythm with a short PR interval and delta waves most prominent in lead V4 (arrows). There is a relatively tall R wave in leads V1 and V2. These findings suggest the diagnosis of WPW type A syndrome.

37a

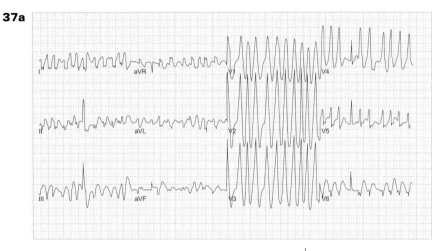

37b

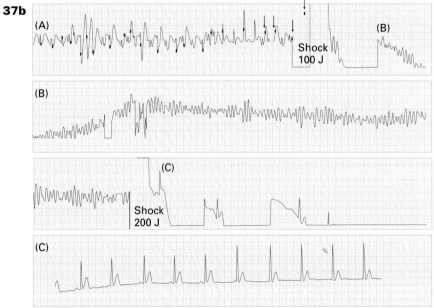

37c

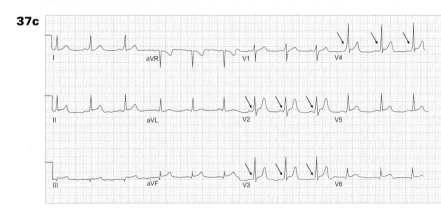

Question 38

A 62-year-old male presented with fatigue, dizziness, and worsening congestive cardiac failure.

1 What are the findings in **ECG 38a** and what is the underlying cardiac rhythm?
2 What does **ECG 38b** show?

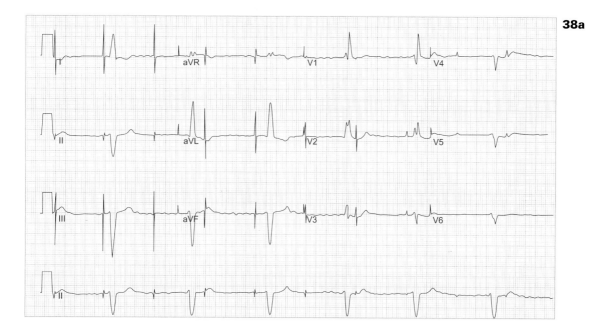

38a

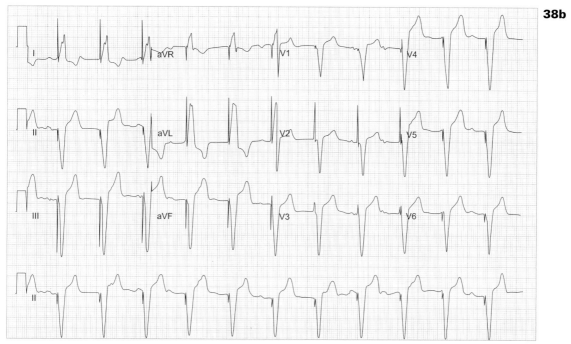

38b

Answer 38

1 ECG 38a shows a failed single chamber (VVI) pacemaker. There are pacing potentials (arrows) that are not followed by a QRS complex showing an absence of ventricular capture. There are no P waves visible and no atrial pacing potentials. This underlying ECG shows the presence of atrial fibrillation with fairly regular and broad abnormal QRS complexes at a rate of 36 bpm, indicating complete heart block on a background of AF.

2 In contrast to the previous ECG, **ECG 38b** shows a single chamber ventricular pacemaker that is functioning normally. This is characterized by the presence of AV asynchrony where there is no relationship between the presence of the P waves (arrows) and the broad QRS complexes preceded by a pacemaker spike. Therefore, there is no atrial sensing or pacing and the pacemaker is of the VVI type.

38a

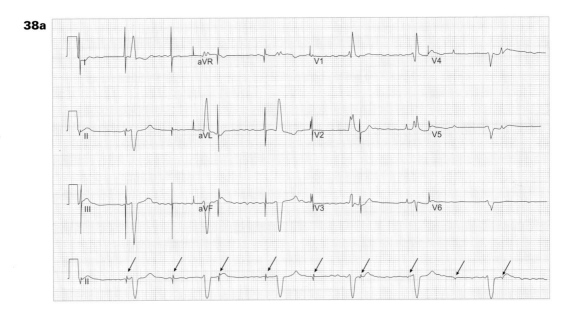

38b

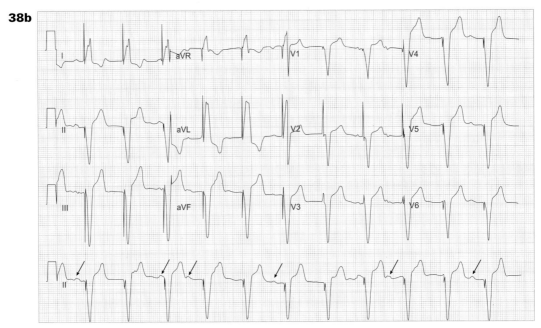

Question 39

A 56-year-old male presented with the symptoms of palpitations. There is a history of high alcohol consumption and no history of ischaemic heart disease.

1 What are the findings in **ECG 39a**?
2 How can the diagnosis be confirmed?
3 What does **ECG 39b** rhythm strip show?
4 How should the patient be managed?

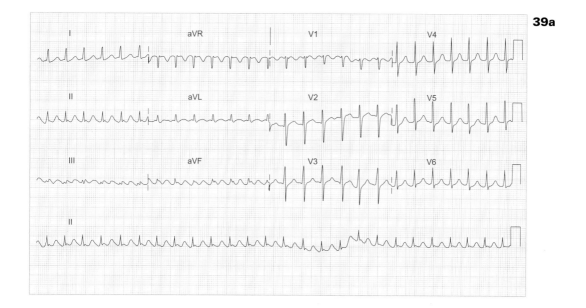

39a

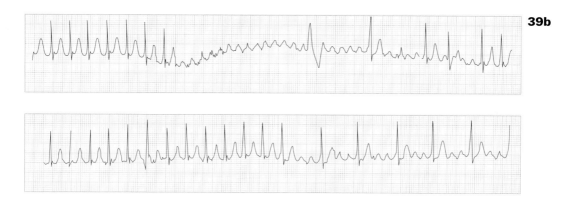

39b

Answer 39

1 ECG 39a shows narrow complex regular tachycardia with a heart rate of 156 bpm. There is evidence of P wave activity best seen in the rhythm strip (arrows). This ECG shows SVT. The differential diagnosis is between an atrial flutter, AV or AV nodal re-entrant tachycardia.

2 The diagnosis can be confirmed by increasing the AV block by manoeuvres such as carotid sinus massage, valsalva manoeuvre, or by administering adenosine. The increased AV block would allow flutter waves to become prominent, thus helping in the diagnosis. Adenosine can terminate the nodal re-entrant tachycardia. The increased AV delay results in a slower ventricular rate. However, it has side-effects such as severe bronchospasm and chest tightness and many patients may not tolerate it. It should be avoided in patient with a history of severe asthma.

It is important to note that carotid sinus massage is contraindicated in patients with carotid bruits, a history of ventricular fibrillation or VT, MI, transient ischaemic attack, or stroke in the last 3 months. Continuous ECG monitoring and resuscitation facilities should be available when conducting this procedure.

3 ECG 39b shows the powerful effect of carotid sinus massage. Carotid sinus massage stimulates the vagus nerve, thus enhancing the block at the AV node. The increased AV block has made the atrial flutter waves very prominent. The carotid sinus massage resulted in transient complete heart block with a ventricular escape beat (broad QRS complex beat; circle) followed by normal narrow complex beats.

4 The management of atrial flutter is similar to AF. Underlying risk factors such as ischaemic heart disease, thyroid disease, rheumatic heart disease, and cardiomyopathy should be investigated. The usual investigations include U&E, FBC, TFT, LFT, CXR, and echocardiography.

The main aims are: ventricular rate control, anticoagulation to prevent thromboembolism, and restoration of sinus rhythm. The ventricular rate control can be achieved by AV node blocking drugs such as digoxin, verapamil, and beta blockers. Heparin can be used initially to reduce the risk of thromboembolism. However, if atrial flutter persists then heparin should be replaced with warfarin as in AF. The restoration of sinus rhythm may be achieved by drugs such as amiodarone, flecainide, propafenone, or sotalol, or by synchronized electrical cardioversion.

39a

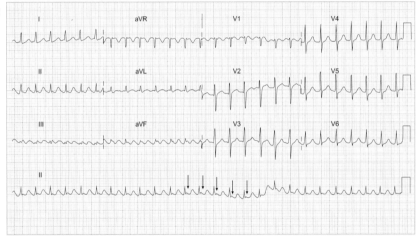

39b

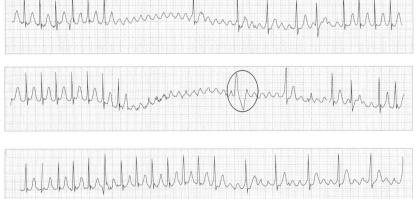

Question 40

A 74-year-old female with a past history of ischaemic heart disease presented with palpitations and light-headedness.

1 What are the findings in **ECG 40a**?
2 What is the differential diagnosis of SVT?
3 **ECG 40b** is taken from another patient. What does it show?

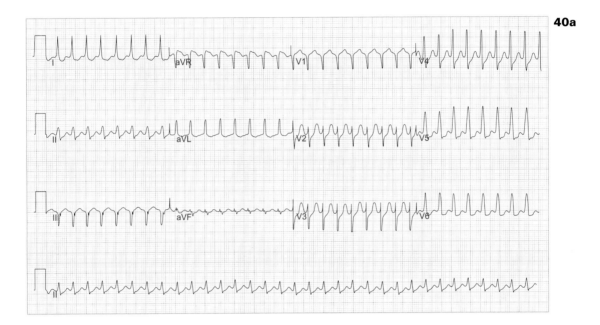

40a

40b

Answer 40

1 ECG 40a shows narrow complex tachycardia at a rate of 200 bpm. There is no clearly defined P wave activity. The QRS complex is of normal morphology. It therefore arises above the bifurcation of the bundle of His and is supraventricular in origin. There is ST segment depression in leads L1, aVL, and V4, V5, and V6.

2 SVT is a term that is usually used to describe tachycardia originating from above the AV junction. This includes sinus tachycardia, atrial tachycardia, and junctional tachycardia. SVT generally appears on the ECG as a narrow complex tachycardia wereby P waves may or may not be visible.

In sinus tachycardia, P waves of normal morphology are visible which precede QRS complexes.

In atrial tachycardia, P waves are usually visible which are of different morphology to sinus rhythm. Atrial rates in focal atrial tachycardia may vary between 150–250 bpm. Varying degrees of AV block may be present. These may be caused by ectopic focal firing or due to localized re-entry. Atrial flutter is a macro re-entrant tachycardia in the right atrium with 'saw-toothed' flutter waves visible on ECG. Atrial rates vary between 280–350 bpm, but typically 300 bpm where 2:1 AV block gives a ventricular rate of 150 bpm. Atrial fibrillation is the commonest sustained arrhythmia characterized by fast irregular atrial activity (rates >350 bpm) with varying AV conduction leading to irregular ventricular rate. Atrial activity may be visible on ECG but not organized P waves.

Junctional tachycardia is re-entrant tachycardia involving the AV node. In AV nodal re-entrant tachycardia (AVNRT), the re-entry circuit is within the AV node with simultaneous activation of both the atria and the ventricles. P wave activity is usually coincidental with QRS complexes and may therefore be 'hidden' or may appear just after the QRS complexes as r' in lead V1 or small S wave in lead V6. In AV re-entrant tachycardia (AVRT), the reentrant circuit is formed between the AV node and an accessory pathway such as the bundle of Kent in WPW syndrome. The retrograde limb of the circuit is usually the accessory pathway with retrograde P waves appearing shortly (but not immediately) after the QRS complexes.

3 ECG 40b is similar to **40a**. However, in this example there is evidence of P wave activity at the end of the QRS complexes best seen in leads V1–V2 and in the rhythm strip (arrows). This suggests AVRT.

40a

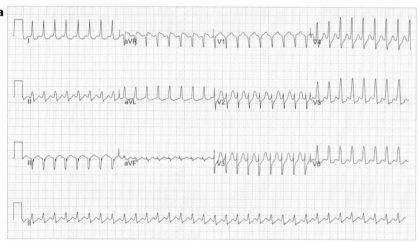

40b

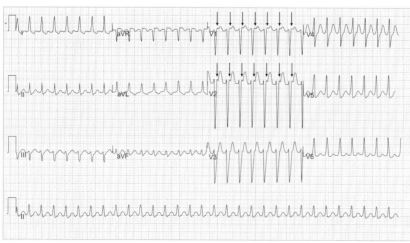

Question 41

A 38-year-old female with a previously known carcinoma of the breast presented with acute shortness of breath. On examination her pulse was 124 bpm and irregularly irregular, with a BP of 84/62 mmHg (11.2/8.3 kPa). Her jugular venous pressure was elevated and her chest was clear.

1 What are the findings in **ECG 41**?
2 What further investigation is required to confirm the diagnosis?

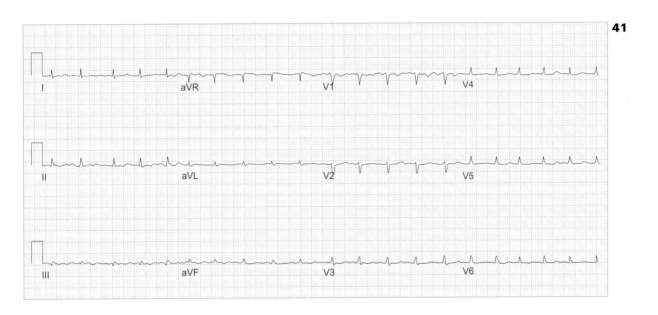

41

Answer 41

1 ECG 41 shows AF with a ventricular rate of about 130 bpm. The axis is normal. The most striking abnormality is the low voltage complexes that are present throughout the ECG. These abnormalities in the context of the clinical findings strongly suggest the diagnosis of a large pericardial effusion and impending cardiac tamponade.

2 The diagnosis should be confirmed by echocardiography. However, other investigations may be required, including CXR, arterial blood gases, and a possible VQ scan or CT pulmonary angiography to rule out the presence of pulmonary embolism. In hypothyroidism and severe obesity, low voltage ECGs can be expected but the clinical presentation would be different.

In this patient a malignant pericardial effusion is highly likely due to her past history of carcinoma of the breast. The diagnosis would be confirmed by cytological examination of the pericardial fluid.

41

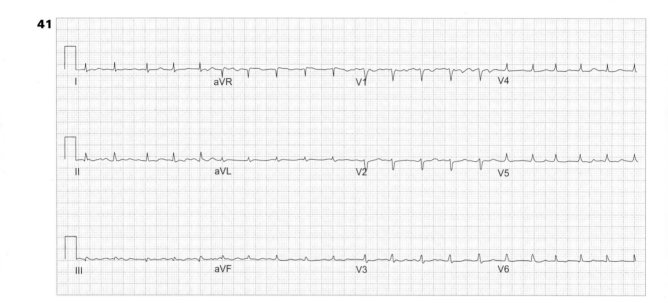

Question 42

An 82-year-old male known to have previous AF presented with a collapse. He was on digoxin, warfarin, and co-amilofruse. On examination his pulse was 40 bpm and BP was 162/60 mmHg (21.6/8.0 kPa). There was bilateral ankle oedema. His jugular venous pressure was not raised and his chest was clear. **ECG 42** was taken in the accident and emergency department.

1 What are the findings in **ECG 42**?
2 What further investigations are required?
3 How should this patient be managed?

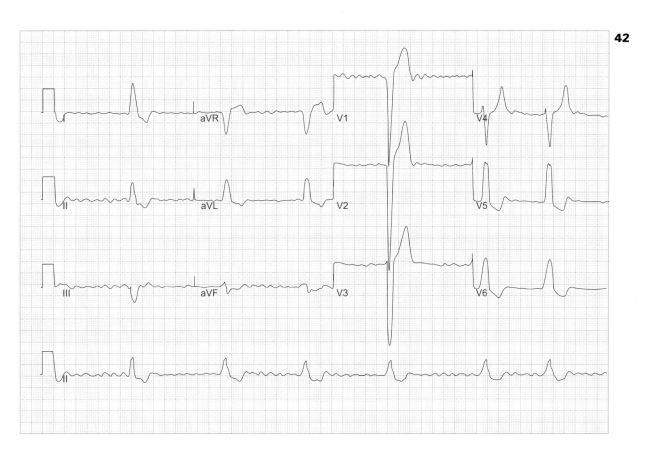

42

Answer 42

1 ECG 42 shows AF with a slow ventricular rate of 39 bpm. There is also LBBB.
2 Further investigations include U&E, FBC, cardiac enzymes, thyroid function tests, digoxin levels, 24-hour Holter monitoring, and echocardiography.
3 The most likely cause for the dizzy spells in this patient is bradyarrhythmia. Digoxin toxicity may have precipitated this. In elderly patients sick sinus syndrome should also be considered. In the further management of the patient, digoxin should be stopped and a further 24-hour Holter should be requested. If it still shows bradyarrhythmia a permanent pacemaker should be considered.

After stopping the digoxin it is quite possible that the patient may develop fast AF, leading to worsening of congestive cardiac failure. In such a situation a permanent pacemaker would still be useful to prevent the development of significant bradycardia and, therefore, allowing the use of digoxin and other rate-slowing drugs required for the management of tachyarrhythmias. The use of warfarin should be carefully assessed, especially if there is an ongoing relative contraindication.

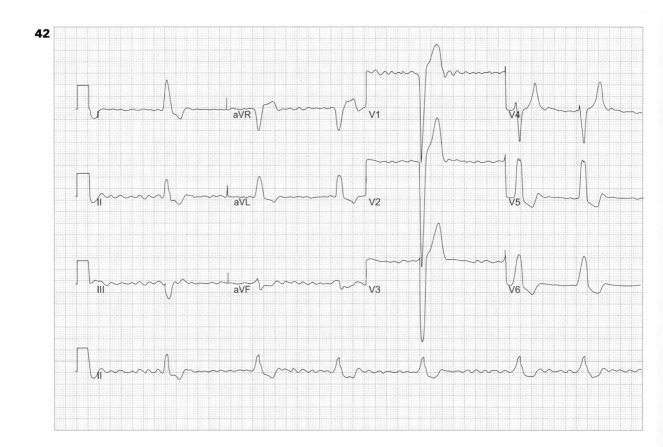

42

Question 43

A 44-year-old female with known pernicious anaemia presented with a history of weight loss, anxiety, and intermittent palpitations. She had an Hb of 10.5 g/dl (105 g/l) and an MCV of 102 fl. **ECG 43** was performed on her admission.

1 What are the findings in **ECG 43**?
2 What single investigation is required to confirm the diagnosis?

43

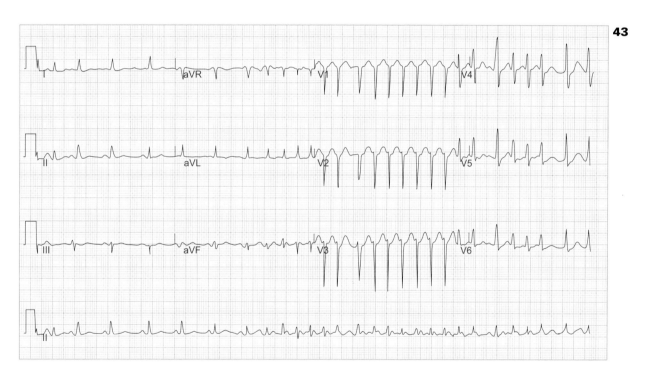

Answer 43

1 ECG 43 shows sinus rhythm in the initial part. There is a normal axis and no other significant abnormalities. The rhythm strip of the ECG shows sinus rhythm in its initial seven complexes. The eighth complex (arrow) is an atrial ectopic beat as evidenced by a different P wave morphology. This atrial ectopic has led to the development of AF in the remaining part of the rhythm strip. These findings suggest the diagnosis of paroxysmal AF. A 24-hour Holter monitoring should be requested to assess the frequency of paroxysms.

2 Thyroid function tests (free T3, free T4, and TSH) should be requested to confirm the diagnosis of hyperthyroidism. In this patient the presence of thyrotoxicosis was confirmed. The coexisting pernicious anaemia suggests an autoimmune aetiology.

43

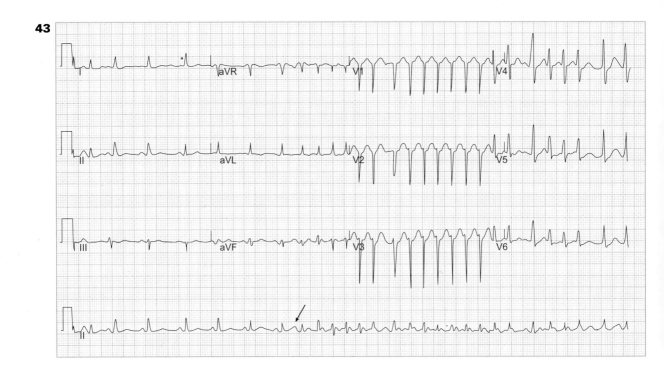

Question 44

A 45-year-old male factory worker involved with heavy mechanical work was found to have **ECG 44** during a routine checkup.

1 What does **ECG 44** show?
2 What is the significance of this condition?

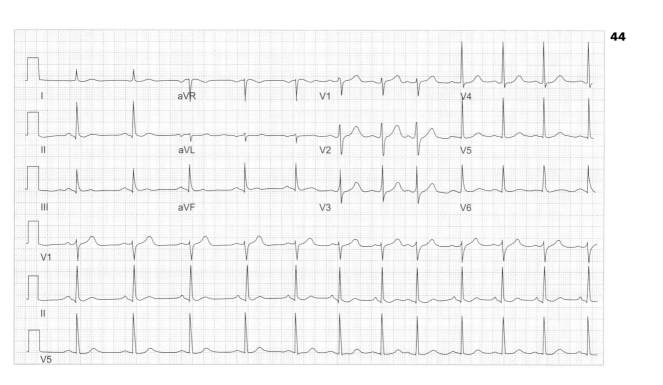

44

Answer 44

1 ECG 44 shows sinus rhythm with a normal axis. There is a continuous variation in the PP interval (markers), most obvious in the rhythm strips. The P wave morphology does not change. There are no other abnormalities noted. The diagnosis is sinus arrhythmia. The differential diagnosis includes atrial ectopics and SA block. Atrial ectopics can be differentiated by varying P wave morphology. SA block can be differentiated by an abrupt change in the rhythm.

2 Sinus arrhythmia is a benign condition and does not have any clinical significance. It is commonly found in athletes, people who do heavy mechanical work, and in children.

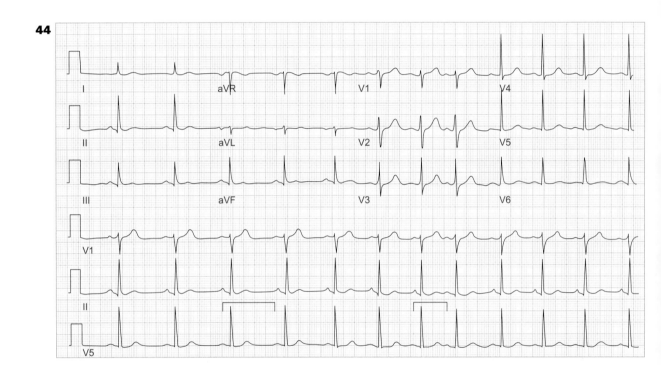

Question 45

A 34-year-old female with a history of recurrent sinusitis and infertility was found to have **ECG 45**.

1 What are the findings in **ECG 45**?
2 What is the differential diagnosis?
3 What is the association of this condition?

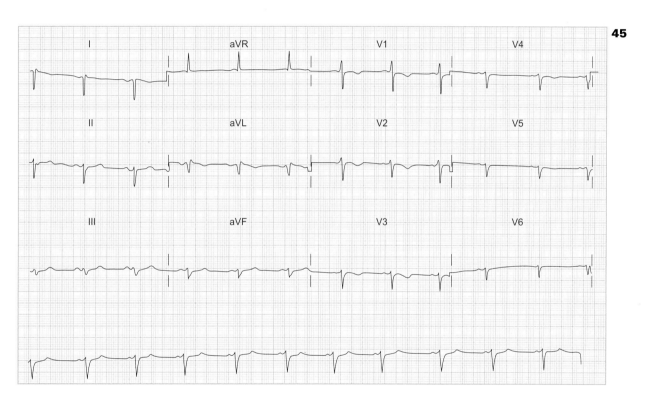

45

Answer 45

1 ECG 45 shows sinus rhythm with an extreme right axis deviation (RAD). The P wave is upright and R wave is tall in lead aVR. There is a deep S and flattened T wave in lead LI. The height of the QRS complexes gradually decreases from leads V1–V6. The chest leads show a right ventricular pattern with a small R and deep S wave in leads V5 and V6. There is also T wave inversion in leads V1–V3.

2 The differential diagnosis is either dextrocardia or improper electrode position with transposition of the right and left arm electrodes. The abnormalities in improper electrode placement are limited to the limb leads. Since the changes in the ECG are also noted in the chest leads, the most likely cause for the abnormality is dextrocardia. This was confirmed on CXR.

3 Dextrocardia may be associated with Kartagener's syndrome. Other features of Kartagener's syndrome include recurrent sinusitis, bronchiectesis, situs inversus, and male infertility. It is due to defective motility of the cilia lining the respiratory epithelium and of sperm. Kartagener's syndrome is an autosomal recessive disorder.

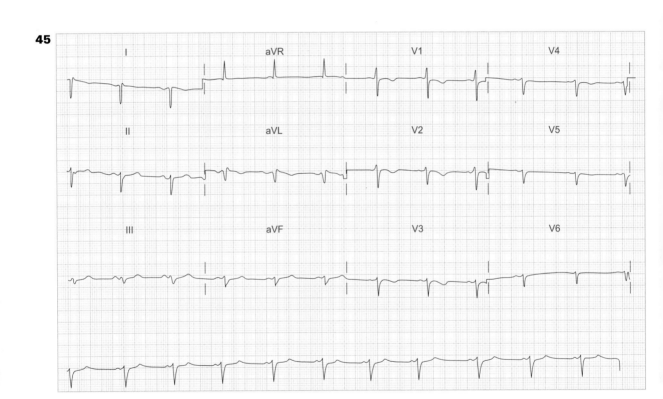

45

Question 46

A 78-year-old male presented with a crushing retrosternal chest pain. He was hypotensive with a BP of 80/60 mmHg (10.7/8.0 kPa). The neck veins were engorged and the chest was clear.

1 What are the findings in **ECG 46a**?
2 What does **ECG 46b** show?

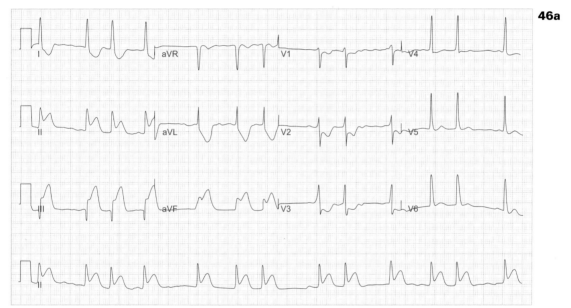

46a

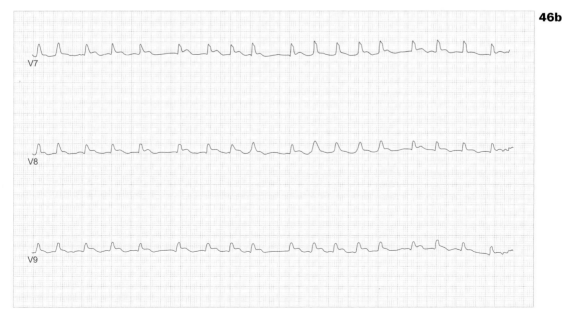

46b

Answer 46

1 ECG 46a shows an irregular rhythm due to AF. There is ST segment elevation in leads LII, LIII, and aVF, and ST segment depression with T wave inversion in leads LI and aVL (arrows). The leads V1, V2, and V3 show ST segment depression and a relatively tall R wave (circles). The diagnosis in this ECG is acute inferior wall MI with lateral wall ischaemia and posterior wall extension.

2 ECG 46b shows the posterior leads V7, V8, and V9. All these leads show ST segment elevation (arrows) confirming the presence of posterior wall MI. One can deduce the presence of acute posterior wall MI from a conventional ECG by finding a tall R wave and ST depression in leads V1 and possibly V2. The R wave is the reciprocal of the Q wave in the posterior leads. The ST segment depression is the reciprocal of the ST segment elevation accompanying the acute infarction.

46a

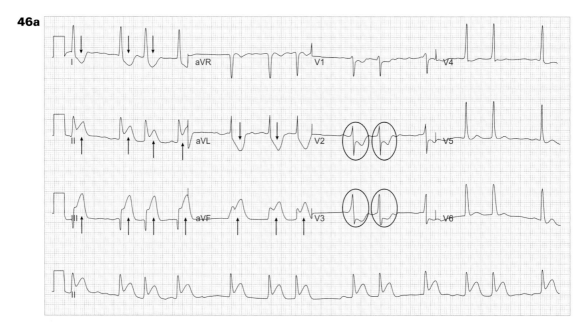

46b

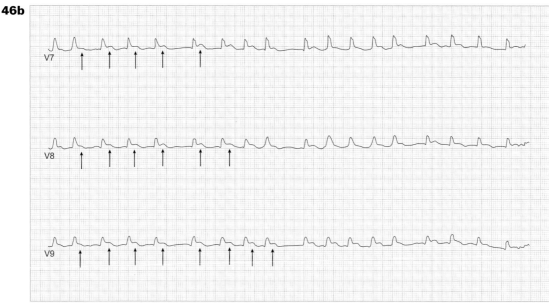

Question 47

A 74-year-old male with a history of renal failure was admitted with progressive drowsiness. He had a history of hypertension and was found to have a BP of 200/110 mmHg (26.7/14.7 kPa). He was taking co-amilofruse and lisinopril. **ECG 47a** was taken immediately on admission and **ECG 47b** was taken after treatment.

1 What are the abnormalities shown in both ECGs and what is the likely cause?
2 How should this patient be managed?

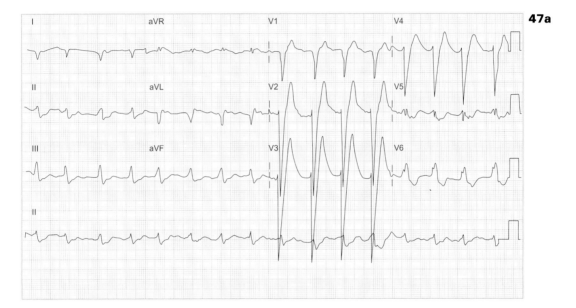

47a

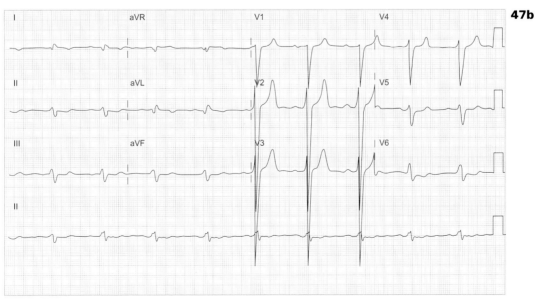

47b

Answer 47

1 ECG 47a shows RAD (170°). P waves are difficult to recognize. The RR interval is regular and QRS complexes are broad, with an M-shaped pattern in V6 as in LBBB (arrows). The T waves are tall and peaked (tented T waves; arrows), seen especially in leads V1–V3. In the context of the clinical history the most likely cause for these abnormalities was hyperkalaemia. In fact the serum K+ on admission was 7.9 mmol/l (7.9 mEq/l). **ECG 47b** was taken after treatment when the serum K+ had dropped to 6.4 mmol/l (6.4 mEq/l). There is sinus rhythm with clearly visible P waves and a prolonged PR interval (264 ms). The axis is normal and the LBBB appearance in **ECG 47a** has also disappeared. The QRS complexes are less broad and there is a reduction in T wave amplitude which still remains peaked in V2–V3 (arrows). The changes are consistent with resolving yet residual hyperkalaemia. Other changes seen with hyperkalaemia include junctional escape rhythm and severe broadening of QRS complexes eventually resulting in ventricular fibrillation.

2 The emergency treatment of hyperkalaemia depends on the ECG changes. It should be considered as an emergency in the presence of such changes. Immediate calcium gluconate infusion should be given, followed by insulin and dextrose infusion. More definitive treatment later on includes calcium resonium. In this particular case co-amilofruse and lisinopril should be withheld and alternative antihypertensive agents considered.

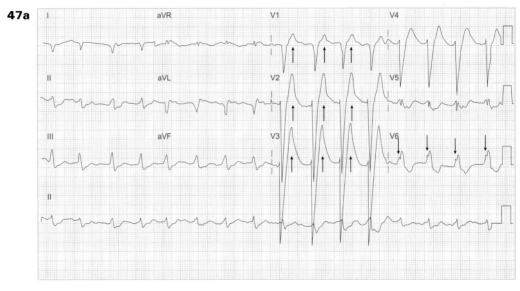

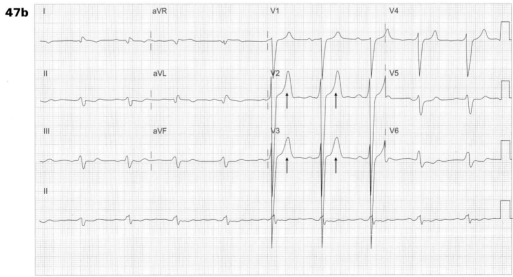

Question 48

A 37-year-old female who was partially deaf presented with palpitations.

1 What abnormality is shown in **ECG 48** and what is the significance?
2 What further advice needs to be given to the patient?

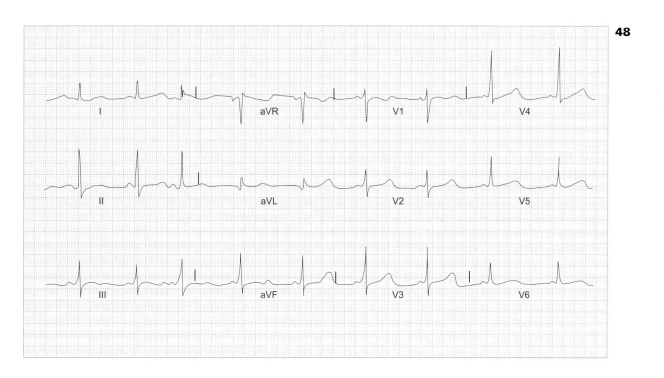

Answer 48

1 ECG 48 shows normal sinus rhythm. The most prominent abnormality is a prolonged QTc of 570 ms (marker). A prolonged QT can be hereditary or acquired. It can lead to development of life threatening ventricular arrythmias such as torsades de pointes and ventricular fibrillation. This can result in sudden cardiac death.

Two varieties of the hereditary form have been reported. The Jervell and Lange-Nielsen syndrome is associated with deafness, while the Romano–Ward syndrome is not. Both of these disorders are autosomal recessive. While some patients remain asymptomatic throughout life, others are highly susceptible to arrhythmias, particularly torsades de pointes. Patients at high risk of sudden cardiac death are characterized by deafness, female gender, syncope, and documented arrhythmias. The acquired form of prolonged QT may be due to drugs, electrolyte abnormalities, hypothermia, and central nervous system injury. Acquired prolonged QT intervals also carry a risk of serious arrhythmias unless the causative factor is corrected.

2 These patients may benefit from an implantable cardiac defibrillator (ICD). Advice should be given to avoid possible precipitating factors especially drugs that can be bought over the counter such as antihistamines. Screening of family members for the condition is also required.

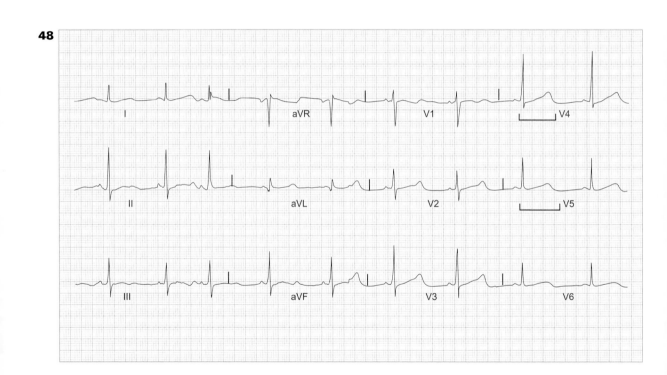

48

Question 49

A 65-year-old male was admitted with acute inferior wall infarction. While in CCU he had a sudden collapse and the arrhythmia in **ECG 49** was noted.

1 What are the abnormalities in **ECG 49**?
2 How should this patient be managed?

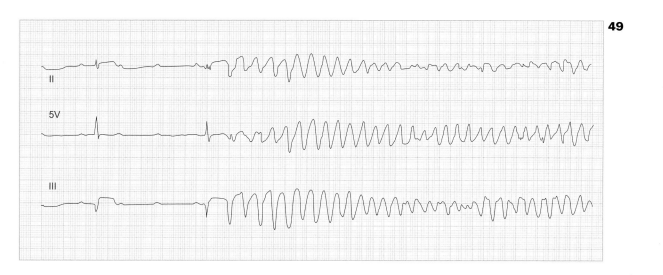

49

Answer 49

1 ECG 49 is a three lead rhythm strip showing complete heart block in the initial part. After the second normal QRS complex a ventricular ectopic is seen, falling at the end of the T wave (R on T phenomenon; arrows). This has resulted in the development of polymorphic VT (torsades de pointes).

Torsades de pointes refers to VT characterized by QRS complexes of changing amplitude twisting around the isoelectric line, giving a characteristic undulating pattern with a varying QRS axis. It carries a risk of degenerating into ventricular fibrillation and sudden cardiac death. A prolonged QT interval may predispose to such a cardiac dysrhythmia.

2 This patient was being monitored when this event occurred. Immediate unsynchronized electrical cardioversion should be carried out in this situation along with advanced life support. As this patient has complete heart block an urgent temporary pacing is recommended. Temporary pacing can help to avoid recurrence of the arrhythmia by increasing the heart rate and shortening the QT interval. An isoprenaline infusion may act in a similar manner.

49

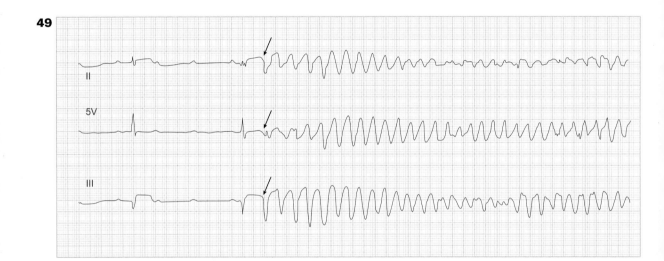

Question 50

An 85-year-old female was brought in collapse into the accident and emergency department. She was found to have a BP of 100/55 mmHg (13.3/7.3 kPa) and a pulse of 150 bpm. **ECG 50a** was performed on initial assessment.

1 What does **ECG 50a** show?
2 The patient was given adenosine intravenously. What does the rhythm strip **ECG 50b** show?
3 How may adenosine help in the management of cardiac arrhythmias?

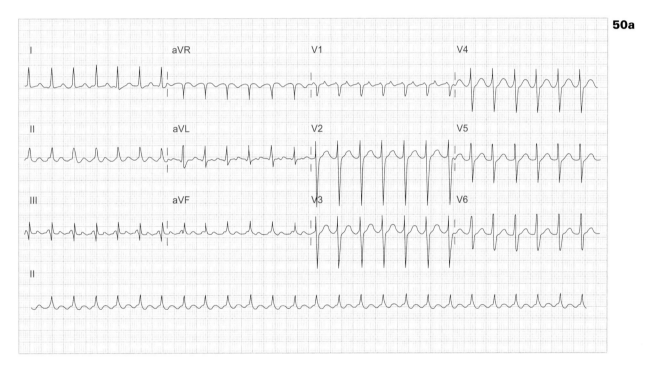

50a

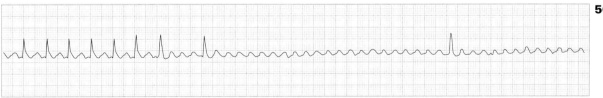

50b

Answer 50

1 ECG 50a shows an atrial flutter with 2:1 block. There are two P waves (arrows) for every QRS complex. Some of the P waves can be seen as small deflections superimposed on the T wave (lead V1).

2 ECG 50b shows a profound bradycardia with flutter waves prominently visible between QRS complexes, confirming the diagnosis of atrial flutter.

3 Adenosine is a useful drug that can be used to terminate paroxysmal SVT. It has a very short half-life of about 8–10 seconds and, therefore, should be given as a rapid intravenous bolus followed by a saline flush, preferably in a bigger vein in the antecubital fossa. It can cause profound bradycardia and possible bronchospasm and is contraindicated in second and third degree heart block, sick sinus syndrome, and asthma.

Adenosine can also be used to help in the differential diagnosis of broad and narrow complex tachycardias. It has no effect on broad complex tachycardias if they are of ventricular origin. Adenosine slows AV conduction and ventricular rate and this results in enhancing the morphological features of the arrhythmias, thus helping in the differential diagnosis as demonstrated in the rhythm strip in this example.

50a

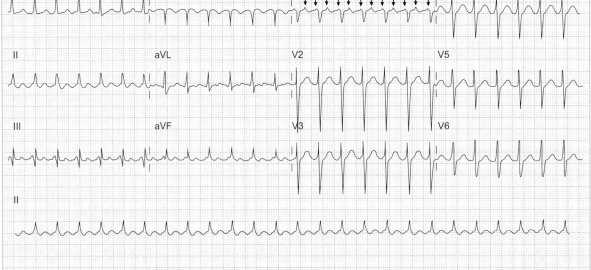

50b

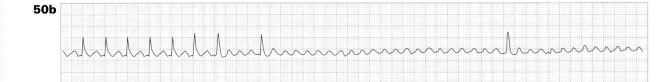

Classification of cases

Index